Taste for life

EAT KINDLY, TREAD LIGHTLY, LIVE WELL

Taste for life

Animals Australia
the voice for animals

ABC
Books

Another world is not only possible, she is on her way. On a quiet day I can hear her breathing.

Arundhati Roy

About Animals Australia

We believe in the power of kindness – in a world where compassion extends to all living beings. Every day, we get out of bed to make that world a reality.

From live animal export to live baiting, puppy farms to factory farms, we are the voice for those who have none. Through investigations, campaigns and public outreach, we inspire individuals, politicians and institutions to make real and lasting change to create that kinder world.

Animals Australia is a team of dedicated staff, volunteers and supporters. Animals Australia is also a team dedicated to good food. Food that tastes good, feels good and does good. Because, creating a kinder world isn't just about big, bold actions. Sometimes it's as deliciously simple as eating consciously and compassionately.

So we hope you'll enjoy these recipes as much as we do and that this book will help you spread a little kindness.

Learn more about our work for animals at: **AnimalsAustralia.org**

Contents

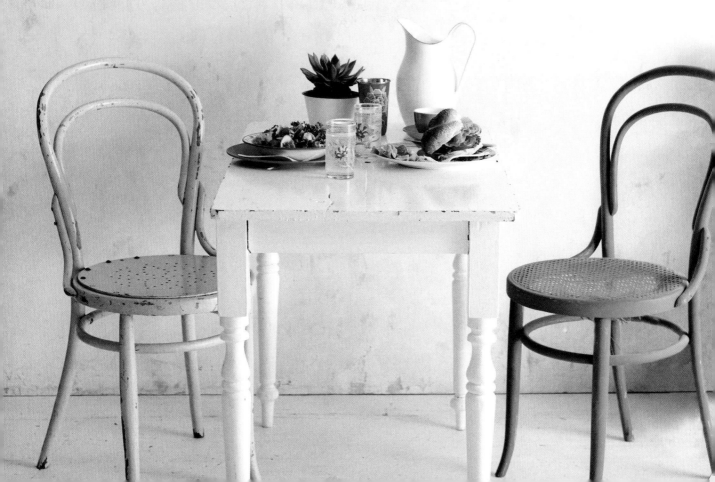

Foreword

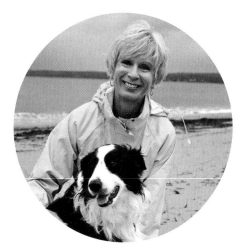

When I told my team that ABC Books had offered Animals Australia the opportunity to write and publish a cookbook the excitement was palpable. After all, there's only one subject that comes up nearly as often as animals in our office, and that's food!

Whether in the lunchroom or sitting around the dinner table at night, food brings people together. It's the glue that binds our days, our traditions and our families. Universally, the preparing and giving of food is a gesture of love. Food does more than fuel our bodies, it nourishes our souls. It defines cultures and customs. In many ways, what and how we eat defines us.

But food has also come to define our relationship with animals – and not in a positive way. I was well into my 30s when I first realised that I was unwittingly part of a system responsible for the systemic and unjustifiable abuse of our fellow species. Of course, I always knew I was eating 'chicken', but I had never stopped to think about the chicken herself. To consider *her* life and whether *her* suffering justified *my* lunch.

I was a fully grown adult when I realised that I had never actually made a decision to eat animals. I simply ate animals because my parents did. And my parents ate animals because their parents did. The realisation that this was an inherited choice, rather than a conscious one, was life-changing for me.

Twenty years on, we are seeing the first stages of a profound paradigm shift. More and more people are consciously thinking about what they eat, realising that the single greatest contribution they can make for the health of our planet, and for our own and our family's health, while also preventing unnecessary suffering, is to rethink the diet we inherited from our ancestors.

This book is a celebration of food and of life. Once you open the doorway to plant-based meals you'll discover a whole world of exquisite tastes and delights.

Enjoy foods that fuel and sustain Olympic athletes, the world's best tennis players and people from all walks of life who are making this shift for a variety of important reasons.

I'm so incredibly proud of our team of advocates who have pulled together this massive project. A huge thank you, also, to the many contributors to this cookbook, from friends and family to a number of very talented chefs who specialise in plant-based cuisine. If the divine smells emanating from our office over the past few months can suggest anything, it's that the tried and tested recipes within these pages are guaranteed to make mouths water and tastebuds sing.

If, like me, you're a creature of habit, then you'll find lots to love in Comfort Food. Don't let anyone ever tell you that you can't make friends with salad! Check out Super Salads for recipes that are sure to impress. If you're just looking for something quick and easy – and very tasty – we've catered for you, too. And if you have a sweet tooth, there are some delicious cakes and desserts to satisfy those cravings.

Taste for Life is so much more than a how-to guide to plant-based food. It's a journey of discovery and one we are thrilled to share with you.

Lyn White

Lyn White AM, Campaign
Director, Animals Australia

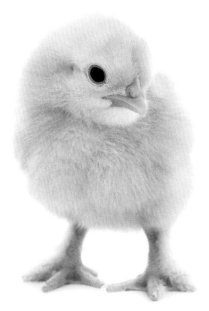

Welcome

~~~~~~~~~~~~~~~~~~~

If you're reading this, you've already taken the first step towards discovering a world of delicious plant-based meals. In your hands is a recipe for good food, great health and a dash of kindness – everything you need to celebrate a *Taste for Life*!

Whether you're simply looking to enjoy more of the fresh fruits and vegies on offer, or you want to reap the benefits of switching to a plant-based lifestyle, we've got you covered. In the pages that follow you'll find a cornucopia of tasty and nourishing dishes and treats.

But this is more than just a cookbook. If you want to live a healthy life ... if you care about the environment ... if you want to protect animals, then this is your guide to putting your values into action.

And you're in good company. Already, one in four Australians are eating less meat in favour of healthy plant-based options.[1] From meat-free Mondays, to part-time vegetarians, to the growing number of vegans – as a nation more and more of us are looking for a more sustainable, cruelty-free and healthier way to live. In fact, Australia is the third fastest growing global market for plant-based products.[2] Millions more people around the world are making similar choices to improve their health, protect animals and care for our planet. By 2041, a quarter of all people living in the UK are expected to be vegetarian.[3] And in the land of fast food and super-sized meals, the stereotypical American diet is also taking a turn for the better, with meat consumption on a steady decline.

Perhaps the best sign that healthy, sustainable eating is here to stay is the huge range of flavoursome plant-based meat, egg and dairy alternatives that are popping up on supermarket shelves everywhere. It's never been more fun, delicious or easy to eat consciously.

And with this book in hand it'll be even easier. You'll discover why greening your diet is kind to animals and the planet, and how loads of health benefits come from eating less meat and more vegies, fruits, grains and pulses. Whether you want to dip your toe in the water or dive right in, we guide you through making the switch, including maintaining proper nutrition, along with some helpful tips.

One in four Australians are eating less meat in favour of healthy plant-based options.

Next, it's time to talk food – starting with your pantry. We cover kitchen staples and introduce you to the delicious array of plant-based alternatives to meat, egg and dairy products. If you have a sweet tooth, there's plenty to explore beyond the fruit and vegetable aisle of your supermarket, as well.

Let *Taste for Life* be a glorious beginning to your tantalising journey into the world of plant-based cooking. Prepare to discover a smorgasbord of mouthwatering meals for all tastes and occasions. Breakfast through dessert and everything in between is covered here, from super healthy soups and salads, to hearty comfort foods, to utterly indulgent cakes and sweets. Within each chapter you'll find recipes you can whip up in a flash as well as dishes that take a little more time – but are well worth the effort!

Feel free to jump around, or take it all in. You might like to start out by cooking one or two new recipes a week. Then, try substituting plant-based ingredients in some of your own favourite dishes. Experiment, explore, have fun and make sure to share the delectable experience with family and friends.

Food is wonderful! With the right ingredients, it can bring people together, nourish our bodies, heal our planet and, of course, taste amazing!

So, fire up the barbie, turn on the oven and join us to eat kindly, tread lightly and live well. Enjoy!

The Animals Australia Team

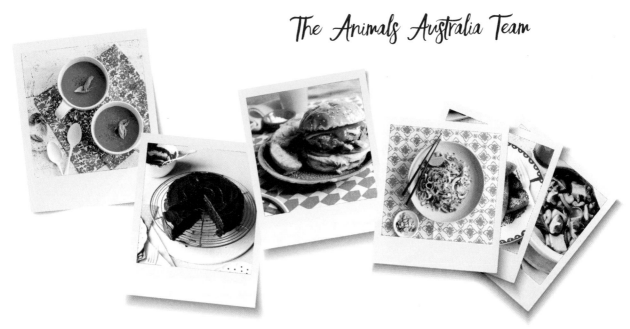

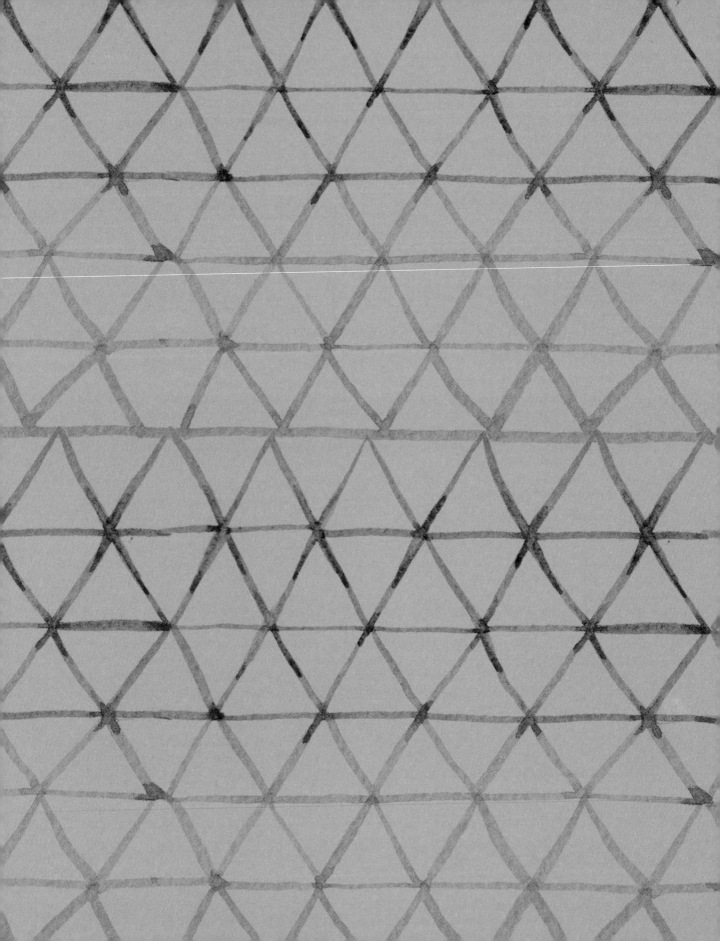

Part One

Food for Thought

Take a few seconds to flick through the recipes in this book and you'll see how mouthwatering plant-based food can be. But there's much more to this story – and it'll make you savour those meals all the more.

From doctors to environmental scientists, animal welfare specialists to economists, experts are coming to the same conclusion – replacing meat, eggs and dairy with plant-based foods can have a profoundly positive impact.

Whether you want to lighten your waistline or your carbon footprint, protect your health or animals – discover how choosing meat-free food is a pathway to a healthier you, a cleaner planet and to sparing countless animals' lives.

Live well

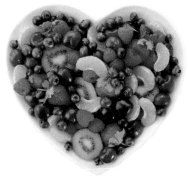

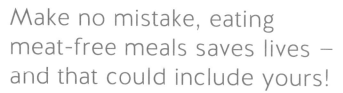

Make no mistake, eating
meat-free meals saves lives –
and that could include yours!

Who doesn't want to live a longer, healthier life? It could be as simple and inexpensive
as treating yourself to plant-based cuisine.

Many people are now realising that eating more foods from plants, and less meat, eggs and
dairy is one of the easiest ways to increase life expectancy and minimise the risk of stroke,
obesity, heart disease, diabetes and cancer – some of the leading causes of death in Australia.
Here are just some of the ways you'll be doing yourself and your family a favour by replacing
animal products with healthy plant-based foods.

LIGHTEN UP

Obesity is at epidemic proportions. Two-thirds of Aussie adults[4] and one in five children[5] are
overweight or obese. Heavy news, right? It gets worse. Obesity is associated with cardiovascular
disease, diabetes, cancer, depression and other chronic diseases.[6] We're eating ourselves to an
early grave. But here's the good news: many people report shedding extra kilos and experiencing
higher energy levels when they cut down on meat, eggs and dairy. In fact, studies have found that
vegetarians and vegans have lower rates of obesity, and are on average up to 20 per cent lighter.[7]
Unlike dairy, eggs and meat (including fish and chicken), plant-based foods such as fruits,
vegetables, nuts and grains are generally low in saturated fat and contain zero cholesterol.

LOVE YOUR HEART

The biggest killer in Australia isn't smoking, drugs or car accidents. It's heart disease[8], which
is directly linked to what we eat. In short, a diet heavy in animal products and low in fruit and
vegies is a passport to ill-health. The saturated fat and cholesterol in animal products can clog
your arteries, placing added strain on your heart. A large-scale study by Oxford University
found that being vegetarian may cut your chances of hospitalisation or death due to heart
disease by 32 per cent.[9]

DODGE DIABETES

As the meat consumption and waistlines of Aussies have grown in recent decades, so has the
rate of diabetes. Type 2 diabetes is now the fastest growing chronic disease in the country.[10]

Quite simply, the more you substitute plant foods for animal foods, the healthier you are likely to be.

Dr T Colin Campbell, nutrition expert at Cornell University

Fortunately, a low-fat, plant-based diet can improve insulin sensitivity, assist weight loss and reduce blood sugar and cholesterol levels – all factors that help prevent and manage diabetes.[11] Whole grains, legumes, fruits and vegetables tend to be high in complex carbohydrates and dietary fibre, which has a positive effect on the metabolism to lower blood sugar levels.

HELP PREVENT CANCER

Few Aussies haven't been affected by cancer, either directly or indirectly. An estimated one in two Aussie men and one in three Aussie women will hear the words, 'You have cancer,' by the age of 85.[12] Luckily, you can improve your odds with what you put on your plate. Research suggests that up to a third of cancer cases are diet related – that's greater than the number of cancer cases linked to smoking.[13]

The World Cancer Research Fund rates processed meats as a group 1 carcinogen, alongside cigarettes and asbestos. And they aren't mincing words: 'The evidence is that whether you are talking about bacon, ham or pastrami, the safest amount to eat is none at all.'[14] Speaking of mince, they also say red meat is 'probably carcinogenic for humans'.[15]

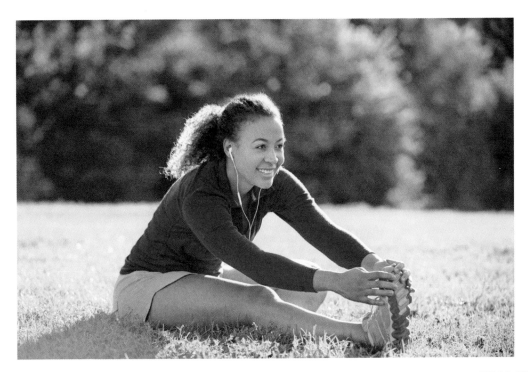

In contrast, fruit and vegetables are generally high in protective antioxidants, fibre and phytochemicals, and whole grains are another excellent source of dietary fibre. So, stack your plate and the odds in your favour with plenty of vegies.

STOP SUPERBUGS

Imagine a world without effective antibiotics – a future where commonplace illnesses, injuries and infections could once again become fatal. Don't freak out, though, we're not there yet. But the World Health Organization, the Food and Agriculture Organization, and the World Organisation for Animal Health have all warned that overuse of antibiotics in animal agriculture risks leading us in that direction.[16]

The overcrowded, unhygienic conditions on factory farms are breeding grounds for disease. Picture this: 'Meat' chickens living and lying for weeks on ground covered in their own faeces. Mother pigs locked in crates, with no choice but to urinate and defecate in the same space they nurse their piglets. Farmed fish swimming in water teeming with parasites and so fouled that it makes it hard for them to breathe. So, animal industries feed farmed animals lots of antibiotics, often even when they're not sick.[17] More than half of all antibiotics produced globally are fed to farmed animals[18] – and this dramatically increases the risk that antibiotic resistant superbugs could develop and spread in human populations. [19]

FORGET FOOD POISONING

Here's where things get gross. Slaughtering animals is a messy business, and we're not just talking about the killing bit. To turn living animals into packaged meat, slaughterhouse workers need to remove their intestines. When faeces from the intestines splashes onto meat, it often contaminates the meat with bacteria that can cause food poisoning.[20] And it's alarming how often this happens. According to Food Standards Australia New Zealand, an estimated four out of five portions of raw chicken meat in Australia are contaminated with faecal bacteria.[21]

The Australian Department of Health's list of high risk foods for food poisoning is a who's-who of animal products: chicken, duck and other poultry; fish and shellfish; raw meat products, dairy products; eggs and egg products.[22] Unlike animal products, most fruits, vegetables and nuts can be safely eaten fresh or cooked.

~~~~~~

If you want to look your best, feel your best and live a long and happy life, then choosing healthy plant-based meals is going to stack the odds in your favour. Not only can you get everything you need to thrive from plants, there's a whole world of delicious cuisine to enjoy.

The benefits of reducing or cutting out animal products extend beyond your own life – it can help our whole community. That's because the treatment of diet-related diseases can put enormous strain on relationships, quality of life and personal budgets – not to mention our national healthcare system.

And it just so happens that when we look out for our own health, we are also looking out for the health of the planet.

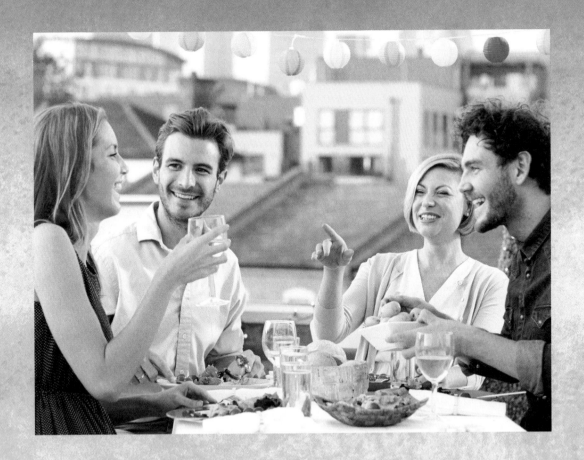

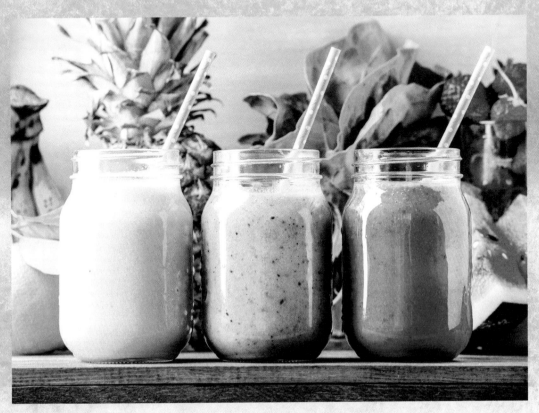

Tread lightly

With our fork we wield the power to create a cleaner, greener planet.

Most of us would agree that if we want our planet to sustain life for generations to come, then we need cleaner energy – to fuel our cars, our homes and our cities. But what about the energy we use to fuel our bodies? Turns out, this may be the biggest problem of all.

Here's the issue: animals eat more food than they produce – an average of six times more.[23] We're feeding huge volumes of edible grains to animals, and then we're eating those animals. It's a bit like filling your car's petrol tank by throwing a bucket of fuel at it: you'll lose more than you gain and make a big mess in the process.

The United Nations (UN) has singled out animal agriculture as 'one of the most significant contributors to today's most serious environmental problems', including global warming, loss of fresh water, rainforest destruction, spreading deserts, air and water pollution, acid rain, soil erosion and loss of habitat.[24]

Fortunately, there's a simple solution: plant-based foods require less land, fossil fuels, water and other resources. Here's how choosing the veg option can help the planet:

HALVE YOUR GREENHOUSE GAS EMISSIONS

Let's cut the bull. No really – cow burps and farts are generating serious emissions that are heating up the planet. Raising animals for food contributes more to global warming than all of the world's planes, trains and automobiles combined.[25, 26] The methane produced by flatulent cows and sheep is a whopping 25 times more potent than carbon dioxide (CO_2).[27] That means we can drive cleaner cars and switch to renewable energy, but unless we reduce our appetite for meat and dairy, experts are warning that climate change will worsen.[28]

Cutting out or cutting back on animal products like meat and dairy can slash your food's greenhouse gas emissions by as much as half.[29]

STOP SOIL AND WATER POLLUTION

It's more than hot air that's coming out of the livestock industry. To give you an idea, a factory farm with 5,000 pigs can produce as much effluent as a town of 20,000 people.[30] But unlike the sewage treatment in most towns, pig factory farms usually leave their effluent in large open aired 'lagoons'. Experts have warned that this can pollute soil, contaminate underground drinking water and run off into rivers and oceans.[31]

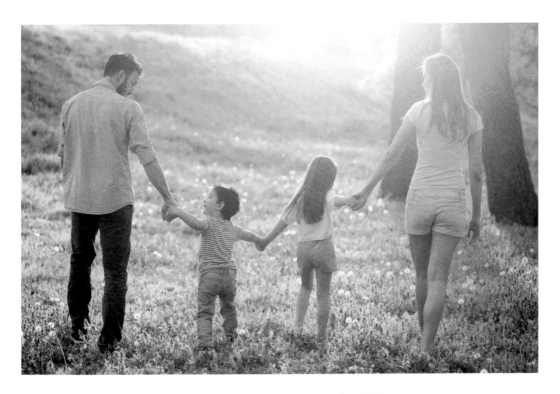

SAVE THOUSANDS OF LITRES OF WATER

For most of us, it's hard to imagine living a day without access to clean water. Unfortunately, for more than one billion people around the world, gaining access to safe water is a constant struggle.[32] And yet, up to one-third of fresh water globally is diverted to meat, egg and dairy production.[33] By contrast, fruits and vegetables require dramatically less water to produce. In fact, by opting for plant-based foods for one week, you can save as much water as if you'd stopped showering for almost six months![34]

HALT HABITAT DESTRUCTION

Our appetite for meat, dairy and eggs is quite literally eating up the planet. Farming animals already uses 30 per cent of the earth's entire land surface and every year vast swathes of forest are bulldozed or burned to graze cattle or grow crops to feed animals in factory farms. Nearly 80 per cent of former forests in the Amazon are now used to graze cattle.[35] Eating meat-free can significantly reduce the amount of land needed to produce your food and in the process protect natural habitats and the animals who live there.

PROTECT OCEAN ECOSYSTEMS

The UN has warned that if we don't reduce current fishing rates, the oceans' fish populations could collapse by 2050.[36] When large trawling nets drag through the ocean they sweep up just about everything and everyone in their path. Alarmingly, often most of the animals who they catch aren't even the animals they're targeting. This 'bycatch' can include dolphins, sharks,

One of the greatest opportunities
to live our values ... lies in the
food we put on our plates.

Jonathan Safran Foer

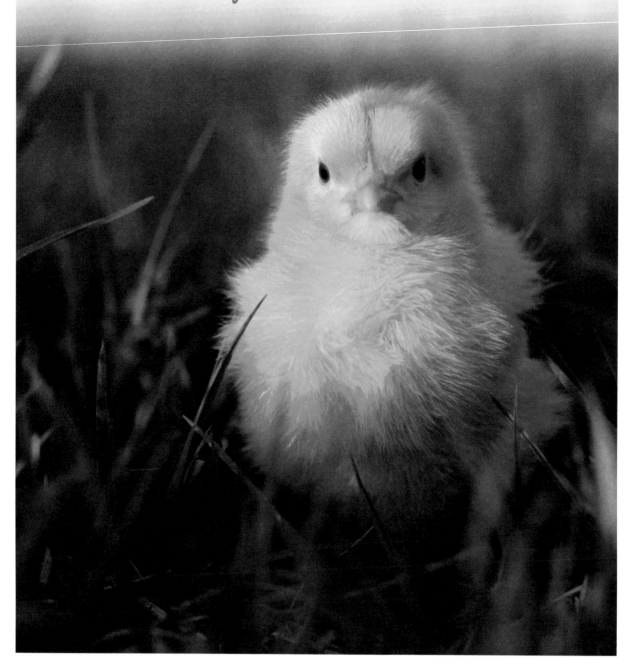

turtles and other threatened species. Prawn trawling is considered the worst culprit. The average prawn trawler tosses back – dead or dying – 80 to 90 per cent of the sea animals they catch.[37]

Fish farming or 'aquaculture' is having a similarly devastating impact. In order to fatten up animals for slaughter, fish farms actually use more fish than they produce. This demand for smaller fish, to use as feed, is leading to even more ocean trawling.[38]

By reducing or replacing the fish and prawns on your plate with healthy plant-based foods you can help let our oceans off the hook – allowing marine ecosystems to recover, and protecting the animals who call them home.

TACKLE WORLD HUNGER

The World Health Organization estimates that one in three people are affected by malnutrition.[39] While many people face a daily struggle to put food on the table, one-third of the world's cereal harvest is being fed to farmed animals.[40] That would be enough grain to feed about 3 billion people. According to Oxfam, 'Increased demand for grains to feed livestock ... is likely to push future food prices further beyond the limits of affordability for the world's poorest people.'[41]

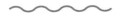

Put simply, making the choice to eat more plant-based foods and less meat, eggs and dairy is not only easy, healthy and affordable, it's also the most powerful way to protect the environment.

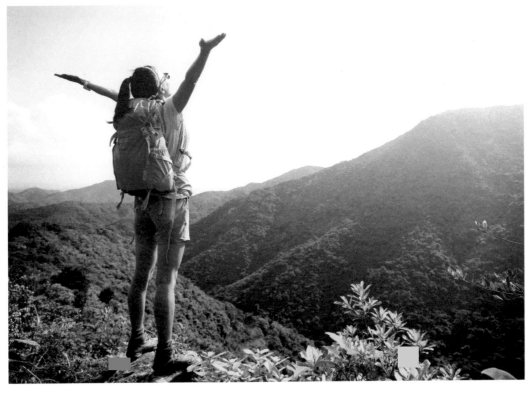

Eat kindly

Every meal is a statement of our values and the kind of world we want to live in.

Sadly, the fairytale farmyards of children's books are just that – a fairytale. The reality for animals used to produce meat, eggs and dairy is far grimmer. Animals in factory farms have their tails, teeth and beaks cut without pain relief. They can suffer in extreme confinement until they are slaughtered. Mother cows suffer separation from their newborn calves so that humans can drink their milk. And day-old male chicks are routinely killed as 'waste products' of the egg industry. While the overwhelming majority of farmed animals live and die in miserable conditions, a lucky few have escaped this fate.

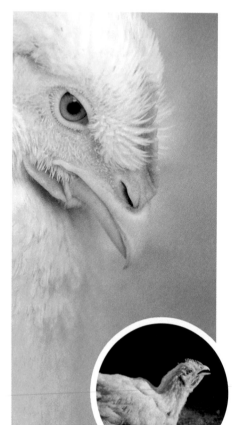

AUTUMN

At just 30 days old, Autumn already carried the weight of an adult hen. Her underdeveloped legs could barely lift her massive body, but when she chirped you could hear she was only a baby. Like all 'meat' chickens, Autumn was born into a body that was designed to produce meat – not sustain life. Inside the overcrowded factory farm she grew up in, many of her companions died from heart failure before they were even six weeks old. Her rescuers knew that she would not survive long after being freed from that windowless shed. But unlike millions of 'meat' chickens before her, Autumn was spared the horror of the slaughterhouse. Instead, her final days on earth were spent bathing in sunshine, eating watermelon and socialising with her BFF (best feathered friend), Summer, at Lefty's Place Sanctuary.

'Meat' chickens are bred to grow so fast that by one month old it can hurt to walk.

Aussie Farms

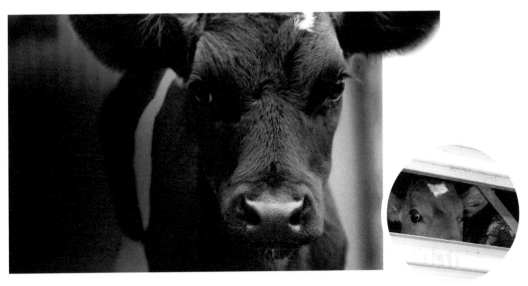

BATMAN

Batman is a gentle, friendly calf who was rescued from a dairy farm at one-day old. Now he lives at Freedom Hill Farm Sanctuary. Every year, hundreds of thousands of baby calves like him are taken from their mothers and killed as 'waste products' of the dairy industry – while their mother's milk is bottled for human consumption.

A dairy cow's calf is normally taken away from her within 24 hours of being born. Mother cows will bellow and call out for their calves when separated.

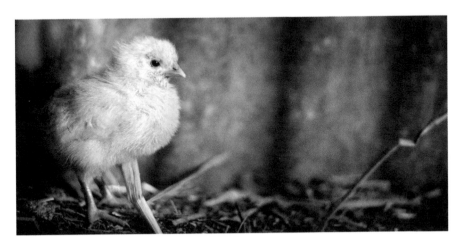

POPEYE

Popeye is an adventurous young rooster, who is very lucky to have hatched at Lefty's Place Sanctuary. If he'd been one of the millions of unwanted boy chicks born into the egg industry each year, Popeye would have been tossed into a mincing machine (alive) or gassed to death on his first day of life.

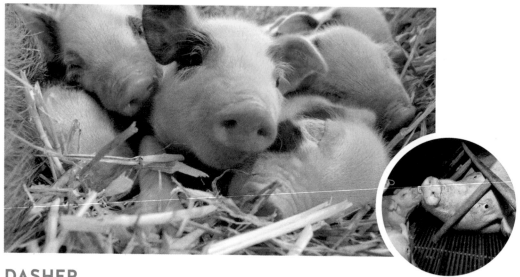

Aussie Farms

DASHER

Born onto Edgar's Mission Farm Sanctuary, Dasher (middle) and his siblings will get to live a full and happy life. Their mother escaped from a pig farm, pregnant, with eight tiny lives inside her. Had she not escaped, Dasher and his siblings would have been trucked to slaughter at just six months old.

In factory farms, mother pigs can spend much of their life in metal crates with barely any room to move.

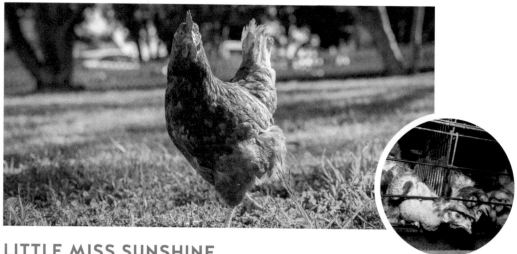

LITTLE MISS SUNSHINE

Little Miss Sunshine comes running when her name is called, loves learning tricks and has even starred in a TV ad. But her life started very differently. Born only to produce cheap eggs, she spent the first 18 months of her life confined to a wire cage. And that's where the story for most egg-laying hens ends. But thanks to the rescue efforts of Edgar's Mission Farm Sanctuary, Little Miss Sunshine has been given a chance to live life to the fullest.

Most hens in the egg industry have the end of their beak cut off without pain relief. And each day, they wake up only to suffer in a tiny metal cage.

FISH FEEL

Did you know that fish communicate with one another, can teach their young, have unique personalities and that many enjoy the company and touch of others? And scientists agree they certainly feel pain.

As commercial fishing trawlers drag sea animals up in large nets towards the water's surface, the change in pressure causes their eyes to balloon out, and often for their swimming bladder to explode. In their last moments, fish gasp and thrash their bodies, slowly suffocating. These trawling nets catch everything in their path, including dolphins, turtles and countless other animals. Other fish are raised in overcrowded, and often disease-ridden factory farms. Recent research has found that fish in fish farms can suffer from such severe stress and depression that they simply 'give up' on life.[42]

WHAT ABOUT 'HUMANE' MEAT?

While the small number of animals raised on small-scale farms may be a little better off than their counterparts on large-scale farms, even these animals may be separated from their families, and often suffer surgical procedures without pain relief. Ultimately both 'factory farmed' and 'free range' animals are trucked to the same slaughterhouses. Investigations have revealed terrifying fates await animals in Australian abattoirs. Find out more at AnimalsAustralia.org/is-meat-humane. (Note: some content contains graphic images.)

ARE 'CAGE-FREE' EGGS A SOLUTION?

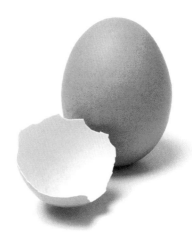

Almost anything is better than the nightmare of factory farming, but sadly, 'cage-free' doesn't mean cruelty-free. The truth is that even on many 'free range' farms, hens spend most of their lives in crowded sheds and may have part of their sensitive beak cut off without pain relief. Across the entire egg industry – including free range and organic farms – chickens are killed from 18 months of age, when their egg production slows. And often, male chicks, who have no commercial value to the egg industry, are gassed or ground up alive on their first day of life.

Since we can live happy healthy lives without harming others, why on earth wouldn't we?

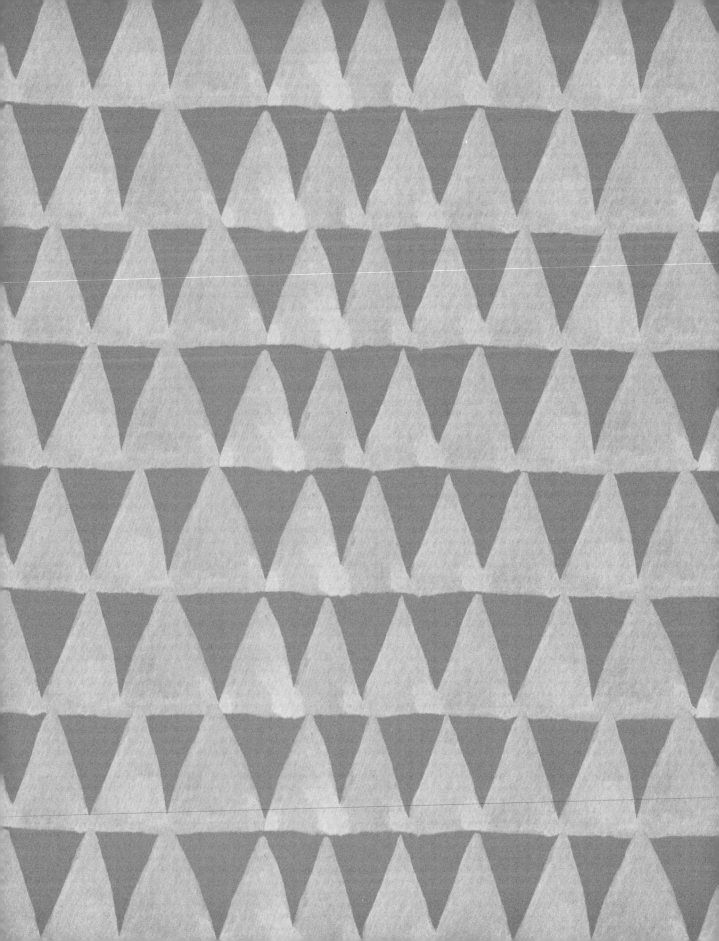

Part Two

~~~

Getting Started

You can get everything you need to thrive
from plant-based foods. And we can show you how.
Protein? Check. Shopping tips? Check. The next few pages
cover all you need to know to take those first few steps
towards your new nourishing and delicious way of eating.

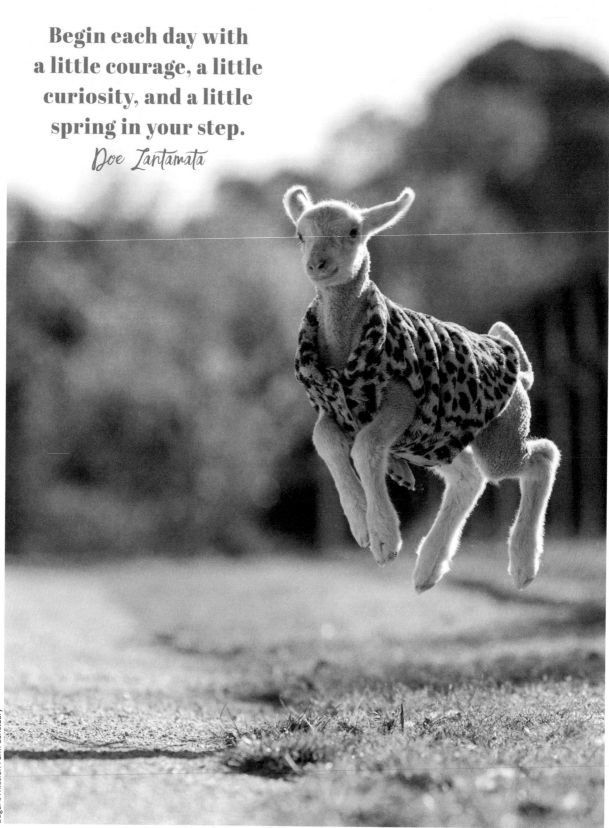

Begin each day with
a little courage, a little
curiosity, and a little
spring in your step.
Doe Zantamata

Take the first step

If you're ready to create a kinder, greener world and care for your body at the same time, here are three simple ways to get started.

START PART-TIME

Cutting out meat doesn't have to be an all-or-nothing decision. For many people, the best way to change their eating habits is to do it gradually. Going meat-free a few days a week, or even for a portion of each day (such as before 6 pm), is a great way to practise compassionate eating, try out new foods and re-invent your favourite dishes using plant-based ingredients. Once you get the hang of it, you can start enjoying even more meat-free meals.

HELP THE MOST ANIMALS

If you're wanting to eat more consciously but aren't ready to go all the way, then start by replacing foods that harm the most animals. More than 95 per cent of the animals we eat and use for food are chickens and fish (plus other marine animals)[43] – and they are some of the most abused animals on the planet. If you begin by replacing chicken, eggs and fish with plant-based options, you can prevent a significant amount of animal suffering.

JUMP RIGHT IN

If you're ready to fully embrace a plant-based lifestyle, then jump in. Make sure to keep it fun, stress-free and easy for yourself – and even better if you have a friend to make the change with you. Keep in mind that it's not about being perfect. So, if you slip up, don't worry. You can always pick up where you left off at your next meal, or try another step suggested here. Finding an approach that works for you is more important than being perfect from day one.

Whichever path you choose, remember that progress is more important than perfection. Every step you take, no matter how big or small, makes a difference. It's far better to eat mostly vegetarian than to do nothing at all. So, celebrate every step, don't stress if you have a hiccup and take it at a pace that works for you.

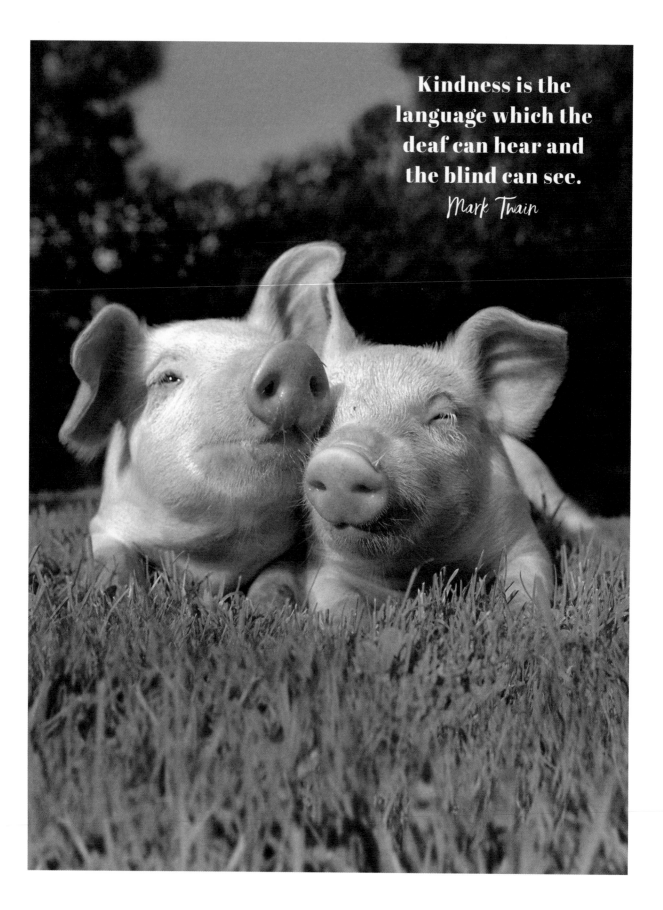

Kindness is the language which the deaf can hear and the blind can see.

Mark Twain

STAYING SATISFIED

Choosing to eat kindly is about giving, not giving up. These simple tips from our team will keep you satisfied and smiling.

LISA: FIND FAMILIARITY

'When I first went vegetarian, I found myself wanting "meaty" meals. But I quickly realised it wasn't meat I was craving. It was the end result: a well-seasoned, sometimes salty, protein-rich meal that was filling and familiar. It didn't take me long to discover that all those elements can be found in plant-based meals that taste just as good – if not better. I now stay satisfied with savoury, filling dishes like sautéed mushrooms, crispy vegetarian meats or a snack of salty mixed nuts.'

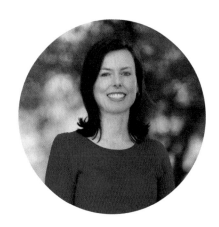

SHATHA: FUEL YOUR BODY

'If you find yourself feeling hungry, you may not be eating enough calories. Because plant-based foods have fewer calories and less fat than animal products, when I ditched meat I found I needed to increase the amount of food I was eating – especially as I lead an active life. I recommend including a variety of foods – plenty of vegies, fruit, grains and seeds and a variety of good fats, which we all need to be healthy. For me, this was a blessing in disguise. Now, I can enjoy more of the foods I love, while maintaining a healthy weight and feeling full of energy.'

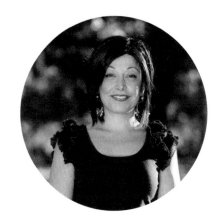

JESSE: DISCOVER DELICIOUS PLANT-BASED PRODUCTS

'I was an avid meat and dairy eater back in the day. I loved a chicken curry, sausage with mash or a toasted cheese sandwich, which is why I was thrilled to discover a smorgasbord of plant-based products that quenched these cravings without the cruelty or saturated fats! From crispy schnitzels and ground 'mince', to creamy dairy-free milk and smooth ice cream, the number of plant-based products has grown massively in recent years, and most supermarkets stock them. My biggest tip is to try a variety and see which ones you like best.'

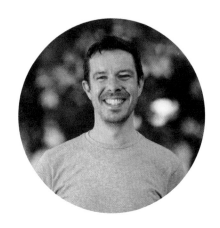

Nourish your body

Here's how you can get what you need to thrive from plant-based foods.

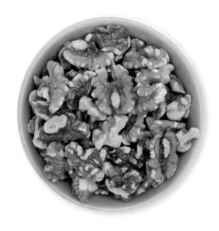

SEEDS AND NUTS

2-3 serves per day

Nuts and seeds are not only a great source of protein and iron, they also support a healthy immune system by providing important minerals and healthy fats. Some of the best sources are peanut butter, flaxseeds, walnuts, almonds, tahini and pumpkin seeds.

1 serve = 30 g nuts, seeds, nut butter or seed butter.

TIP *Grab a handful of almonds as an easy and satisfying snack.*

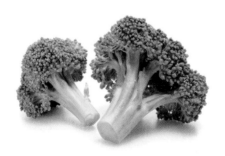

VEGETABLES

5 or more serves per day

Vegetables are some of the healthiest foods on the planet. Some of the most nutrition-packed are kale, broccoli, spinach and capsicum.

1 serve = ½ cup cooked vegetables; 1 cup raw vegetables; or ½ cup vegetable juice.

TIP *Eat the rainbow! The varying, vibrant colours in vegetables exist because of the thousands of healthful phytonutrients.*

Note: These servings act as a guide – the exact daily servings needed will vary based on age, gender, height, weight and activity level. Speak to a qualified health professional knowledgeable about plant-based nutrition for personalised advice.

FRUIT

2 or more serves per day

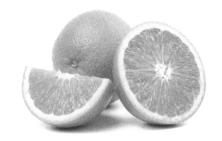

Fruit is great for hydration and a fantastic source of fibre, potassium and antioxidants. Apples, oranges, blueberries, blackberries and bananas are some of the most nutritious.

1 serve = 1 medium-sized piece of fresh fruit or 1 cup cut-up fruit.

TIP *Starting your day with a fruit smoothie is a great way to get your daily servings of fruit.*

GRAINS AND STARCHY VEGETABLES

6 or more serves per day

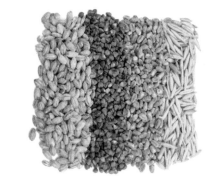

Grains and starchy vegetables are a great source of fibre, iron and protein. Brown rice, pasta, oats and sweet potatoes are a few of the healthiest options.

1 serve = ½ cup cooked rice, pasta or quinoa; ½ sweet potato; ¼ cup muesli; ½ cup cooked porridge; or 1 slice wholegrain bread.

TIP *Whole grains are less processed and more nutritious than refined white grains.*

BEANS AND LENTILS

3 or more serves per day

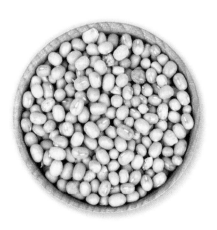

Beans and lentils provide a hefty dose of protein, and many are also a great source of iron and calcium. Kidney beans, split peas and tofu (which is made of soybeans) are some of the best sources. Each day, at least one or two serves should contain a good source of calcium, such as fortified soy milk.

1 serve = 1 cup cooked beans; 170 g tofu; or 1 cup fortified soy milk.

TIP *Always keep a tin of beans handy for salads and snacks.*

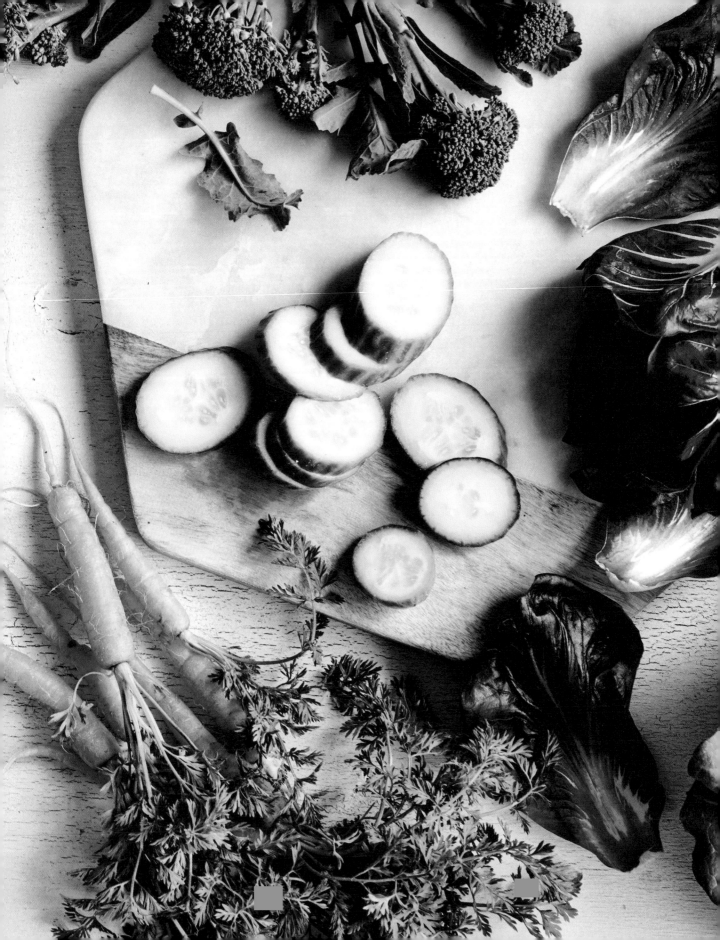

Nutrition 101

Want to take your health to the next level? These four simple tips will have you full of energy and feeling great.

SEEK VARIETY

Getting all the nutrients you need is easy if you eat a wide variety of foods. Fill your plate with foods from every colour of the rainbow. Switch up your meals. And be sure to eat from all of the plant-based food groups: fruit, vegetables, grains, beans and nuts. As they say, variety is the spice of life!

CRUELTY-FREE CALORIES

If you feel hungry or sluggish, you may not be getting enough calories. Sure, vegetables and grains are great, but if that's all you're eating, you may not be giving your body all the fuel it needs. Try adding calorie-rich foods like nuts, seeds, beans, lentils, plant-based meats and healthy oils to your plate, making sure you have a good balance of everything – including protein and iron.

GO GREEN

Leafy greens like kale, spinach and silverbeet are true stars of the vegetable world. They're bursting with essential nutrients, such as calcium, fibre, iron, zinc, iodine and magnesium, plus many B vitamins and vitamins A, C and K. Sauté them with garlic to serve as a side, throw them into your vegie burritos, salads or sandwiches, or blend them into a smoothie for a big daily energy boost.

WHOLE BOWL

Although going meat-free has huge advantages for your health, it's possible to be a 'junk food vegetarian'. After all, cakes, biscuits and chips can all be made without animal products. While it's fine to indulge sometimes, please don't live off chips and soft drink. Be sure you're getting plenty of vegetables, fruit, beans and whole grains in your diet. Your body – and your mum – will thank you!

Protein and iron powerhouses

Want high-quality protein and iron without the saturated fat, cholesterol or cruelty to animals? Dig into these protein- and iron-packed foods.

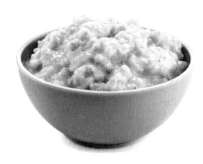

PORRIDGE

A perfect start to a cold winter morning, oats are brimming with iron and fibre to power your day. Vitamin C will help maximise your iron absorption, so add some fresh fruit or drink some juice. Spice it up with nuts, dried or fresh fruit, maple syrup, cinnamon, brown sugar and soy milk.

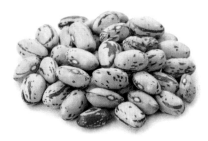

BEANS

Whether black or pinto, kidney or cannelloni, beans are cheap, easy to cook and full of protein. Pop open a tin and stuff them in a burrito, mix them with seasoned rice, toss them through a salad or drop them into a pot of soup – beans can do it all.

LENTILS

Delicious in soups, or with onions and carrots over a bed of rice, lentils are a worldwide favourite. Each serving offers a heap of iron and protein.

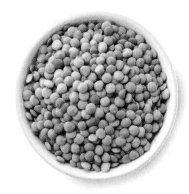

NUTS AND PEANUT BUTTER

Peanut butter on crackers is always a great go-to snack, and nuts can do even more. Adding walnuts, almonds, cashews or other nuts to your cereal, salads and stir-fries is an easy way to add a protein-packed crunch. Or just eat them right out of the packet.

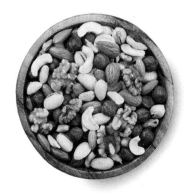

PLANT-BASED MEATS

From burgers to sausages to nuggets, plant-based meats are loaded with protein. They're perfect for quick and easy sandwiches, barbecues and meals that will satisfy even your most carnivorous friends. Check the label before you buy – you want to find products fortified with iron, B12 and zinc, but content varies widely. Some brands are loaded with salt, so beware.

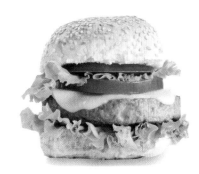

SOY MILK

Great on your morning cereal or in a smoothie, soy milk has as much protein as cow's milk, without the cholesterol. As well as matching the protein content, fortified brands provide similar amounts of calcium so that you're getting this important nutrient, too. Try different brands and flavours to find your favourite.

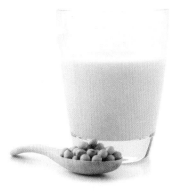

A fit for everyone

Young or old, Olympic athlete or couch potato, a meat-free meal plan can give your body all the fuel it needs to thrive.

According to the Australian Dietary Guidelines and the American Dietetic Association, well-planned vegetarian and vegan diets can not only offer many healthy benefits, they can be appropriate for all ages and life stages.[44] If you have any specific health concerns, or if you are planning a vegan pregnancy or raising a vegan child, seek advice from a qualified health professional knowledgeable about plant-based nutrition. If you're eating an exclusively plant-based diet, it's recommended you take supplements to make sure you're getting enough vitamins B12 and D and Omega-3.[45]

PREGNANCY

Before and during pregnancy, it's recommended that all women take prenatal supplements to get enough essential nutrients, including folate, iron, iodine, B12 and Omega-3. Be sure to eat plenty of protein- and iron-rich foods like beans, lentils, nuts, nut butters, seeds, leafy greens and vegetarian meats. Aim to get a good source of protein at each meal. Iron requirements are quite high during pregnancy and a supplement will help ensure you get enough. Vitamin C can help your body to absorb more iron from your food, so it is a good idea to combine iron-rich foods with fruits or vegetables such as tomato or capsicum. (Avoid having tea or coffee with the meal as these can reduce iron absorption.[46] So can eating a whole lot of bran[47] or taking a calcium supplement with meals.[48]) Omega-3 fats are important for foetal brain development and are found in flaxseeds, walnuts and soy products.[49] You can find folate in green leafy vegetables such as broccoli, spinach, bok choy and salad greens, some fruits, and cereals and breads with added folic acid. Calcium is readily available in tofu, almonds, sesame seeds, tahini, leafy greens (such as kale, bok choy and Chinese broccoli) as well as calcium-fortified plant milks.[50]

BABIES

Breast milk is the best food for babies, and it is essential for mum to get enough additional nutrition during this time. Lactating women need increased amounts of nearly all vitamins and minerals, and extra protein. This can be achieved by eating well and continuing to take a good prenatal supplement, plus additional vitamin B12. If breastfeeding is not possible, a commercial infant formula from a reputable company is the only safe option; check the label for age suitability and always prepare formula strictly according to the instructions.

It is recommended that all mothers of infants on a plant-based diet seek qualified health advice about introducing solids to their baby, as weaning is a crucial time in a baby's development. When starting your child on solids, it is important to continue with breastfeeding or formula to meet nutrient requirements. Make sure your infant is getting plenty of iron from iron-fortified infant cereals, and an iron supplement is also recommended, as well as vitamin B12.

CHILDREN

One of the greatest gifts parents can give their children is healthy eating habits. Introducing children to a whole foods, plant-based diet from the start can set them up with good habits for life. Encourage kids to eat a wide selection of fruit, vegetables, whole grains, nuts, seeds and beans, and to have a good source of protein at each meal.[51]

It is essential to include a source of vitamin B12, for normal growth and development, and healthy blood and nerve function. This can be found in any typical children's multivitamin tablet – and you might also like to grab a B12-fortified soy milk from the supermarket (these often include added calcium as well, bonus!). Brands vary enormously, so check the label to see exactly what you're getting.

Children need a lot of energy and nutrients, but they have small stomachs. Too much fibre can fill them up too quickly and can interfere with the absorption of important nutrients. So, offer your child regular snacks – including a mix of wholegrain and refined grain products, plus fortified soy milk products. Foods high in iron should ideally be combined with a source of vitamin C to optimise absorption.[52]

Make sure children eat calcium-fortified foods and plant milks, plus dark leafy greens such as spinach, silverbeet (Swiss chard), kale and broccoli – whose calcium is actually more readily absorbed than that in dairy. Getting kids to eat calcium from plants also means they're

WHAT ABOUT ...?

CALCIUM: There are plenty of sources of calcium that are kind to cows and don't come with the saturated fat of dairy. Get stuck into soy milk (fortified), sesame seeds, white or brown bread, fortified fruit juice, dried figs, broccoli, green leafy vegetables, molasses, tofu, beans and pulses.

HEALTHY FATS: All fats were not created equal. While the saturated fats in animal products can clog your arteries, there is a host of healthy fats found in plant-based foods. Good sources are nuts, seeds, nut butters and avocados. For Omega-3 fatty acids get your hands on flaxseeds, soybean oil, canola oil, tofu or walnuts.

VITAMIN B12: While it finds its way into animal foods, this bacteria-borne vitamin doesn't get into plants. The good news is that lots of foods, including non-dairy milks, some cereals and nutritional yeast, are now fortified with B12. Even so, if you're eating a plant-based diet, it's a good idea to regularly take a B12 supplement.

Let food be thy medicine and medicine be thy food.
Hippocrates

consuming essential fibre, antioxidants and folate – instead of loading up with the saturated fat, hormones and cholesterol in dairy.[53] If it's a struggle to get your kids to eat their greens, navy beans (such as in baked beans), dried figs and dates, almonds, tahini and sweet potato are all good sources of calcium as well. Blackstrap molasses is delicious on porridge or as a refined-sugar replacement and is full of essential vitamins and minerals like calcium, iron, magnesium, potassium, manganese, copper and selenium.[54]

Here are a few other healthy and delicious snack ideas for kids: vegies cut into fun shapes and served with dip; spread some nut butter on muffins or crackers; fresh fruit; and whole fruit smoothies (rather than fruit juice), which retain all the natural goodness of fibre and phytonutrients – essential for healthy growing bodies and minds!

Keep food simple for young children – complicated unfamiliar dishes can seem daunting to them. For fussy toddlers, having a few tricks up your sleeve can help. Try involving your children in meal preparation. Get them to mash a banana or pour in some of the ingredients. When it's possible to adapt recipe ingredients, let your children help pick what goes into the meal. Children learn by example, so eat what you're feeding your kids – after all, vegies are good for adults, too. Don't give up if at first you don't succeed. It can often be easiest to introduce new foods gradually, and combined with foods your kids already like. And if your children don't like an ingredient in one form, try serving it in another form. For example, if your kids don't like tofu chunks, try using tofu in a creamy dressing; or try mixing grated vegies into pastas or mashed potato.

Teenagers have high energy needs and are often very busy. So, keep plenty of healthy snacks around the house for them. You can also help make social situations a breeze by taking some veg-friendly foods you know your children enjoy to school, parties (check out some kids' party recipes on pages 106–109), sport and other events.

ATHLETES

Because of the high-oxygen and recovery demands of athletes, clean plant-based foods can provide a competitive edge by upping antioxidant and phytochemical intake.[55] If you're training or competing, be sure to consume enough calories to keep your body running at peak performance, and tuck into plenty of high-protein options like plant-based meats, beans, lentils and nuts.

For more information and advice on nutrition visit: **WhyVeg.com/nutrition**

Note: The information contained in this publication is provided for education and information purposes and is not intended to be a substitute for advice or treatment from a qualified health professional. You should seek the advice of a qualified health professional for any personalised dietary advice or health-related dietary assistance.

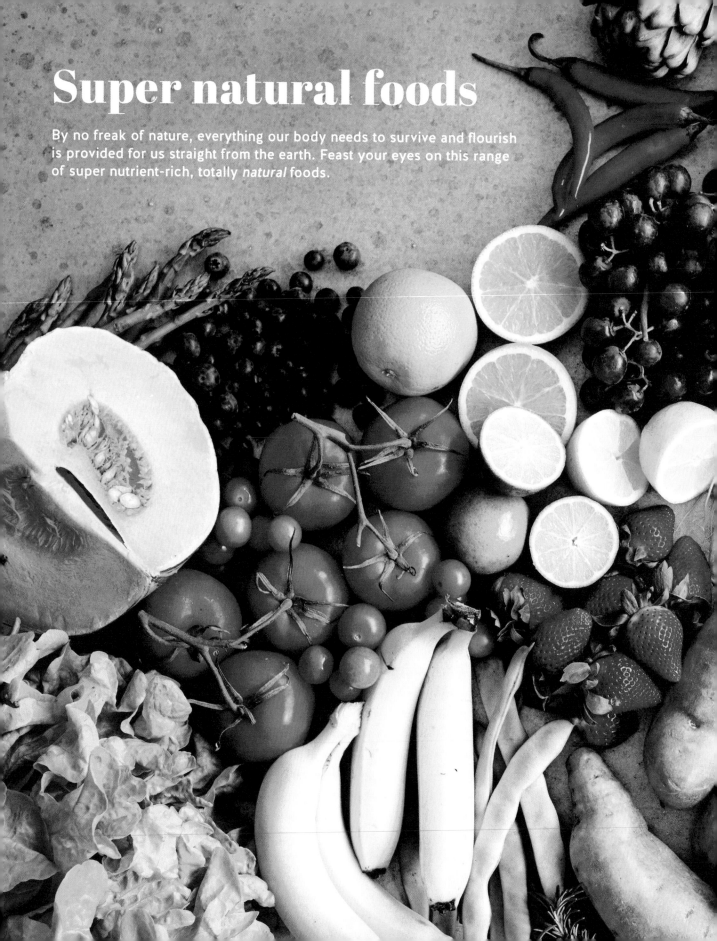

Super natural foods

By no freak of nature, everything our body needs to survive and flourish is provided for us straight from the earth. Feast your eyes on this range of super nutrient-rich, totally *natural* foods.

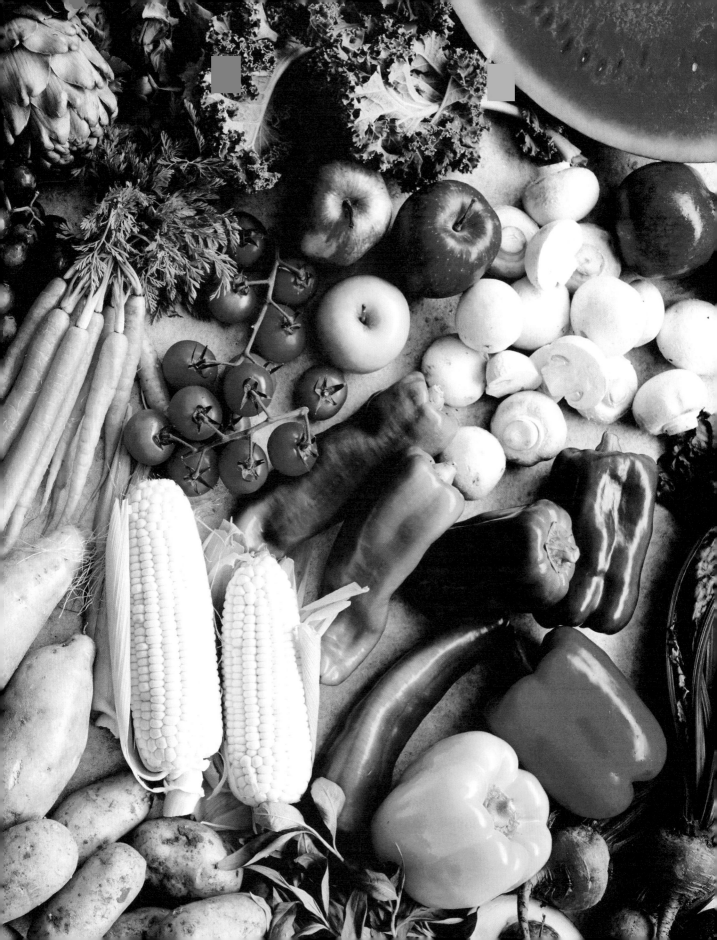

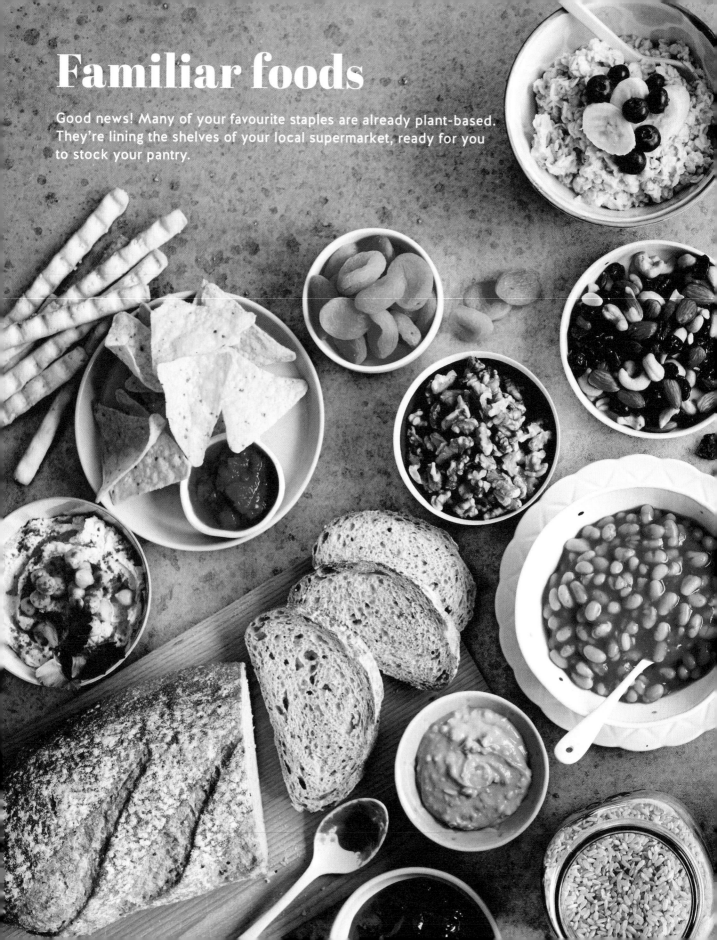

Familiar foods

Good news! Many of your favourite staples are already plant-based. They're lining the shelves of your local supermarket, ready for you to stock your pantry.

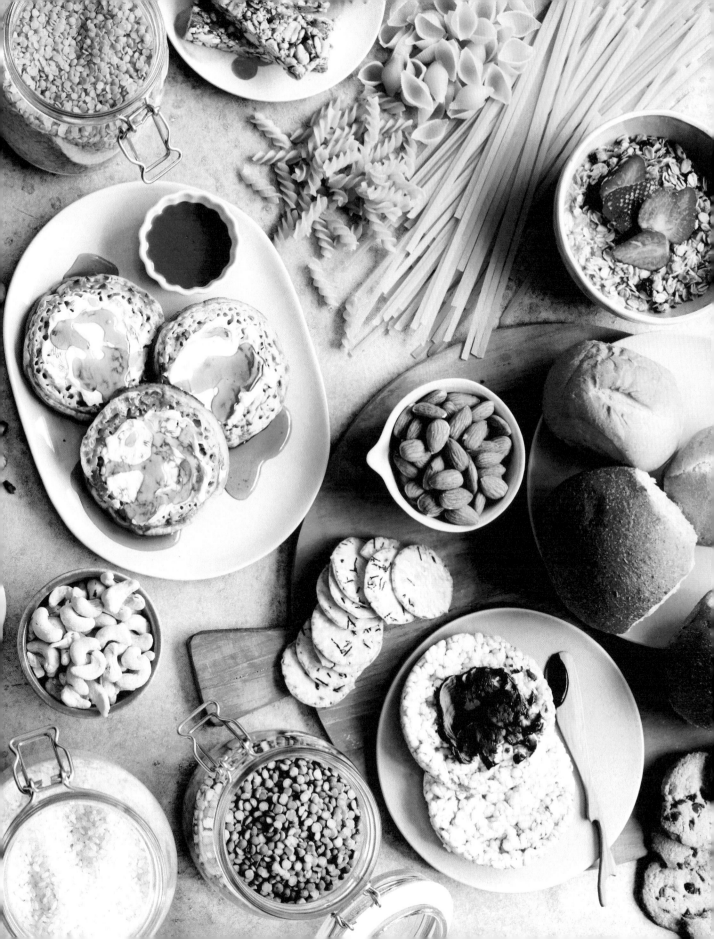

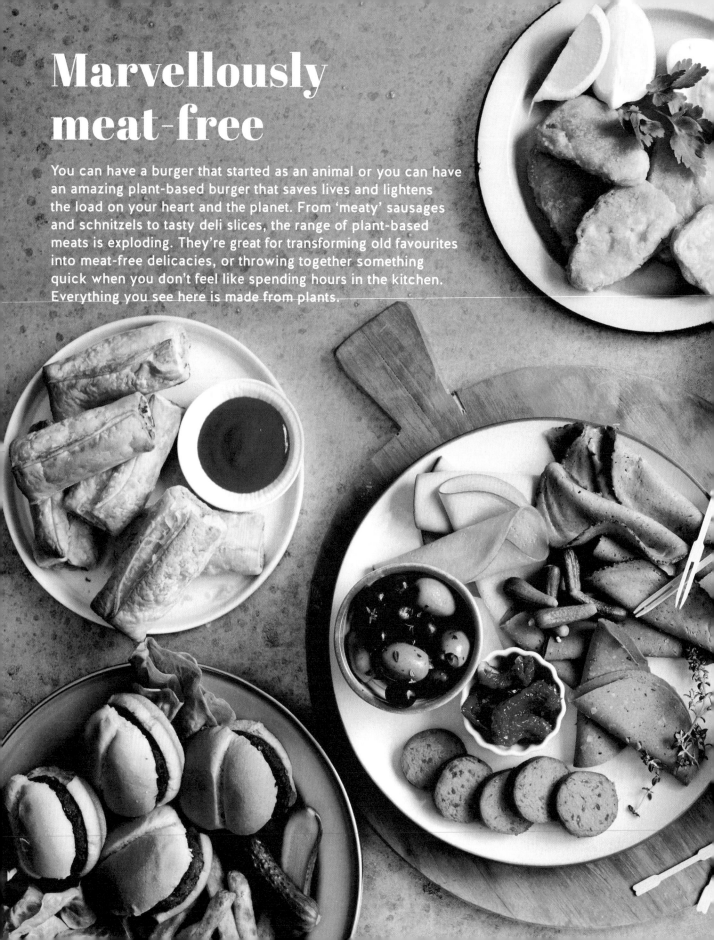

Marvellously meat-free

You can have a burger that started as an animal or you can have an amazing plant-based burger that saves lives and lightens the load on your heart and the planet. From 'meaty' sausages and schnitzels to tasty deli slices, the range of plant-based meats is exploding. They're great for transforming old favourites into meat-free delicacies, or throwing together something quick when you don't feel like spending hours in the kitchen. Everything you see here is made from plants.

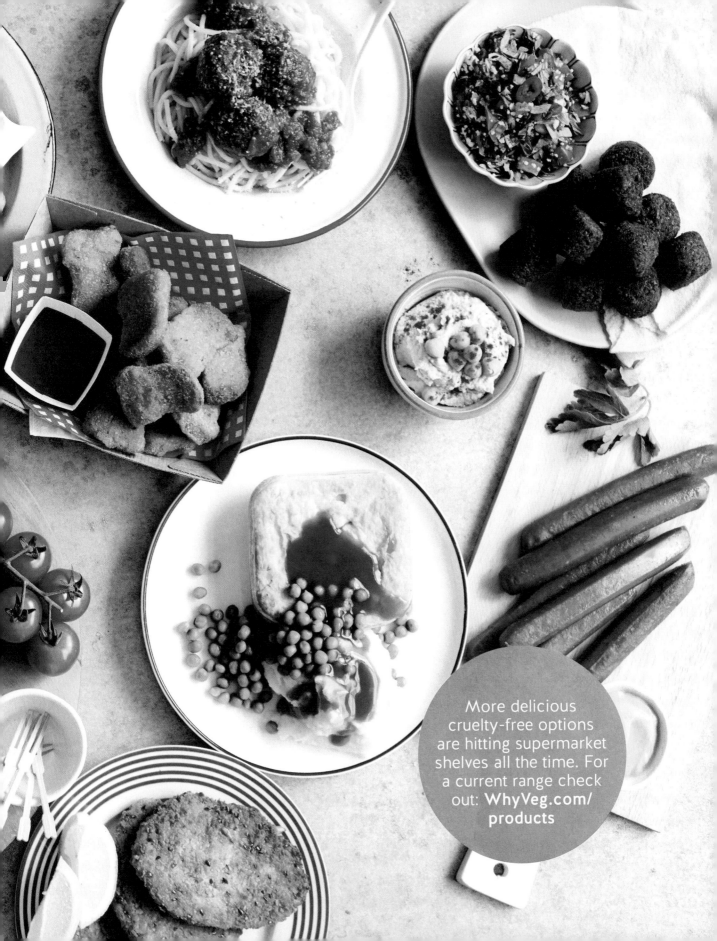

More delicious cruelty-free options are hitting supermarket shelves all the time. For a current range check out: **WhyVeg.com/ products**

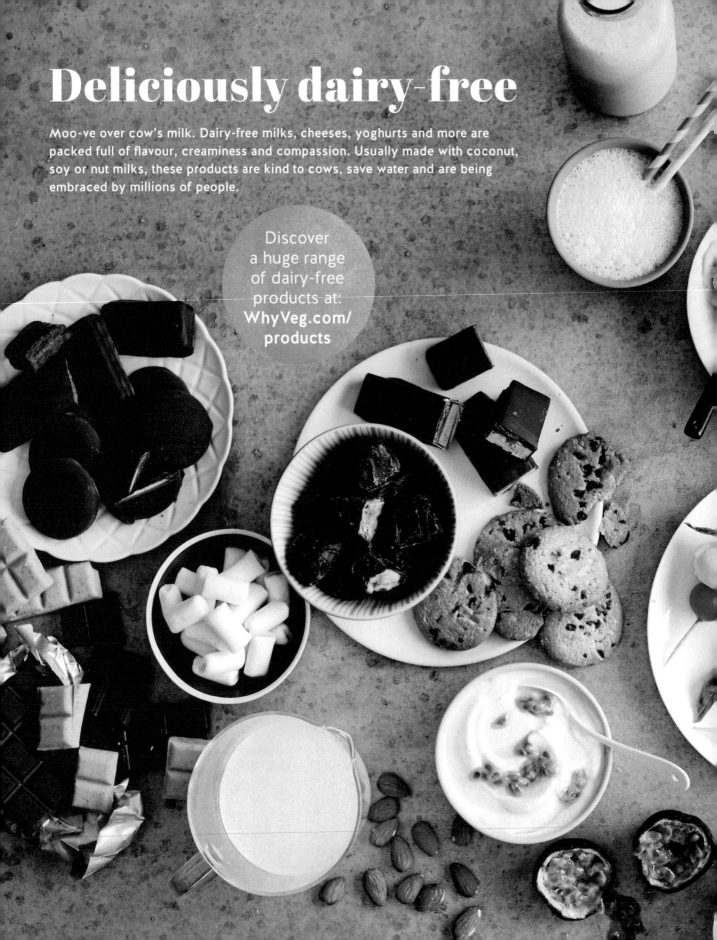

Deliciously dairy-free

Moo-ve over cow's milk. Dairy-free milks, cheeses, yoghurts and more are packed full of flavour, creaminess and compassion. Usually made with coconut, soy or nut milks, these products are kind to cows, save water and are being embraced by millions of people.

Discover
a huge range
of dairy-free
products at:
WhyVeg.com/
products

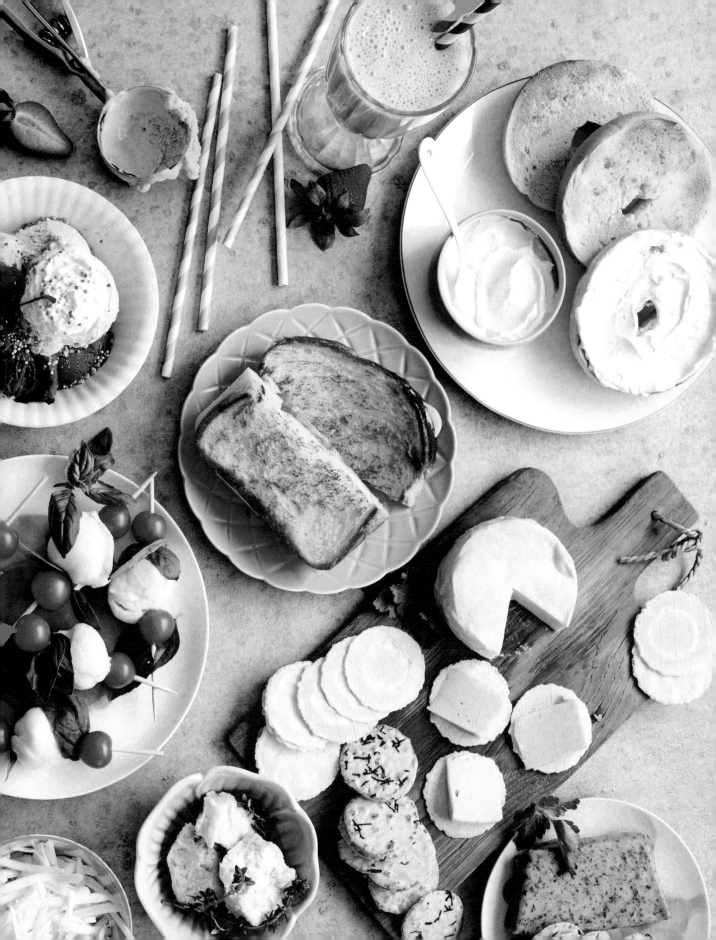

Dinner with friends

Once you've decided to take animals off your plate, how do you handle dinner at a friend's place? And how do you talk about it with family? Don't worry, we've been there, too! These tips will have you covered.

HOSTING THE FAMILY

Serve up traditional meals that you grew up loving and know your family likes – so that nobody feels like they're missing out – but simply make them with plant-based ingredients. Head to pages 164–222 to browse some of our favourite comfort foods and dinners.

DINNER PARTIES

If you're eating at a friend's place, you can help make things run smoothly and stress-free by calling your host in advance and offering to bring a dish or two so that everyone is catered for. The bonus with this plan is that everyone at the dinner will also get to try some of the plant-based meals you love.

SHARE GOOD FOOD!

It's true that the quickest way to someone's heart is through their stomach. Nothing busts myths and sparks positive conversations quite like sharing great plant-based food. Share your favourite dishes with friends and family – and if they ask for the recipe, all the better.

MAKE IT PERSONAL ...

When talking to others about your new way of eating, describe your own reasons for reducing or cutting out meat, in favour of plant-based foods. Be enthusiastic and sincere. Focus on why it excites you and makes you feel good, not on trying to 'convert' people or make them feel bad.

... BUT DON'T TAKE IT PERSONALLY

For some people, the idea of not eating meat can be new and even challenging. The occasional person may find the easiest way to handle this is to joke about it or get defensive. While it's not the response we'd hope for, it's often a sign that your thoughtful choice is challenging them to reflect (possibly for the first time) on their own choices, and sometimes it can take people a little time to process this. So don't take it personally and try not to get defensive.

Offer to discuss things further at another time if they want and then change the subject. And remember, nothing disarms tension better than humour or a joke – even (in fact, especially) when the topic is important to you.

PUT YOURSELF IN THEIR SHOES

Keep in mind that like your family and friends, you once ate meat, too. Not only do you care about your health and the planet, but you're clearly a compassionate person. Approach conversations about vegetarian eating with empathy and patience and try to put yourself in the other person's shoes.

LET THE FACTS SPEAK FOR THEMSELVES

Remember that the facts are on your side. An abundance of evidence shows plant-based eating is better for our bodies, the planet and animals. Don't bury your friends and family with statistics, but if they are interested in hearing more, consider sharing a good book or documentary with them. Why not start with giving them a copy of this cookbook?

Or you could order them a free Vegetarian Starter Kit from **WhyVeg.com/guide**

PRACTISE PATIENCE

Nobody wants to feel judged. If they want to learn more, they'll ask. So there's no need to push the issue. Simply by being a kind and understanding person, you'll open hearts and inspire those around you to make kinder choices over time.

MAKE IT EASY

Make your choice to eat meat-free as easy as possible on the chef in the house. Offer to help with the cooking – after all, you're armed with this book of amazing recipes! You can make meals easier by substituting in vegie burgers, meat-free 'chicken' patties and so on. You can also keep satisfying snacks around the house for when you need something quick, such as muesli bars, tinned soup and nuts.

LISTEN

If your friends or family say they're worried about your health, let them know that you appreciate their concern but try not to get defensive. Share what you've learned about getting proper nutrition and the health benefits of plant-based eating.

BE A ROLE MODEL

Some people will warm to your new lifestyle quicker than others. But stay optimistic. If you're patient with them, and stay healthy and kind, in time they'll come around.

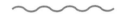

Always remember your choice to eat meat-free is creating a kinder, more sustainable world. That's something you should feel great about!

Eating out

While this book will have you cooking up a storm at home, sometimes you just want a night off. Looking for good plant-based meals when eating out? Global cuisine can be a treasure trove of vegetarian delights.

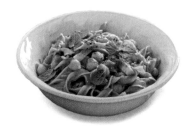

ITALIAN
Vegie pizza hold the cheese (or with dairy-free cheese), pasta primavera, pasta napolitana, risotto, gelato.

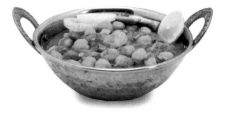

INDIAN
Dhal, vegetarian curries, vegetable samosas, mushroom bhaji, aloo gobi, vegetable dosa, roti.

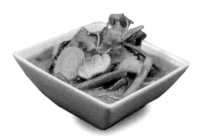

THAI
Pad Thai (hold the egg), vegie spring rolls, rice paper rolls, vegetarian stir-fry – try sweet chilli and basil, lemongrass or cashew dishes.

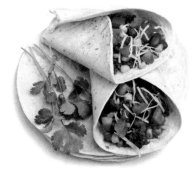

MEXICAN
Bean burrito, taco or nachos without dairy. Jazz it up with extra guacamole.

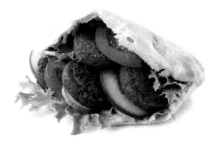

MIDDLE EASTERN
Falafel wrap, hummus, vegetarian dolmades, vegie pide without cheese, Turkish delight.

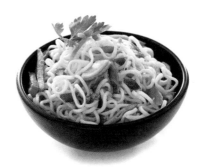

CHINESE
Tofu and veg stir-fries, vegetable dumplings, spring rolls.

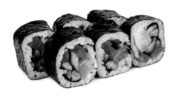

JAPANESE
Vegetable sushi roll, avocado roll, tofu roll, edamame, tempura vegetables, vegetarian udon noodles.

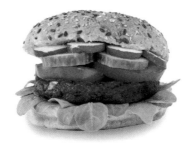

NO-FUSS FAST FOOD
Many cafés and fast food chains you already know also offer plenty of veg options. If you're not sure what's on offer, just ask.

FIND GOOD FOOD ANYWHERE
There's a world of great veg-friendly restaurants to discover, both close to home and just about anywhere on the planet.

To start exploring jump onto: WhyVeg.com/find-me-food

BAM! Build a meal

You don't have to be a master chef to create mouthwatering animal-friendly dishes in the kitchen. With a few simple steps, most of the recipes you already know are probably easy to make meat-free.

SPAGHETTI AND MEAT-FREE BALLS

Fry up balls made with firm tofu or tempeh, onion or shallots, basil and breadcrumbs (see page 169) or buy pre-made ones found in the vegetarian section in many supermarkets.

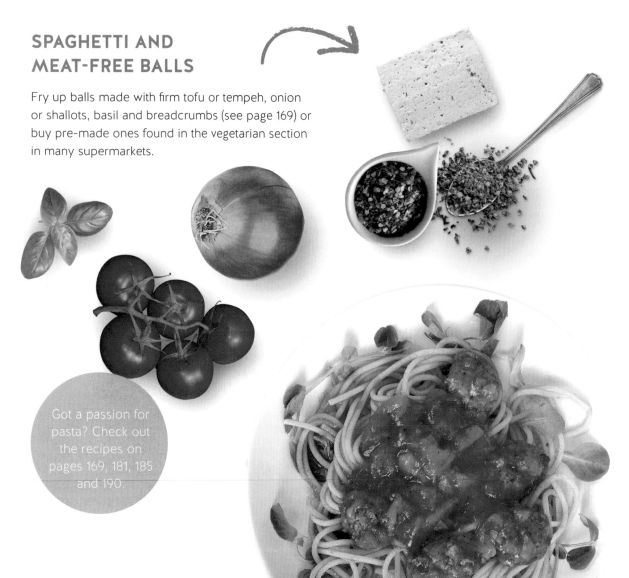

Got a passion for pasta? Check out the recipes on pages 169, 181, 185 and 190.

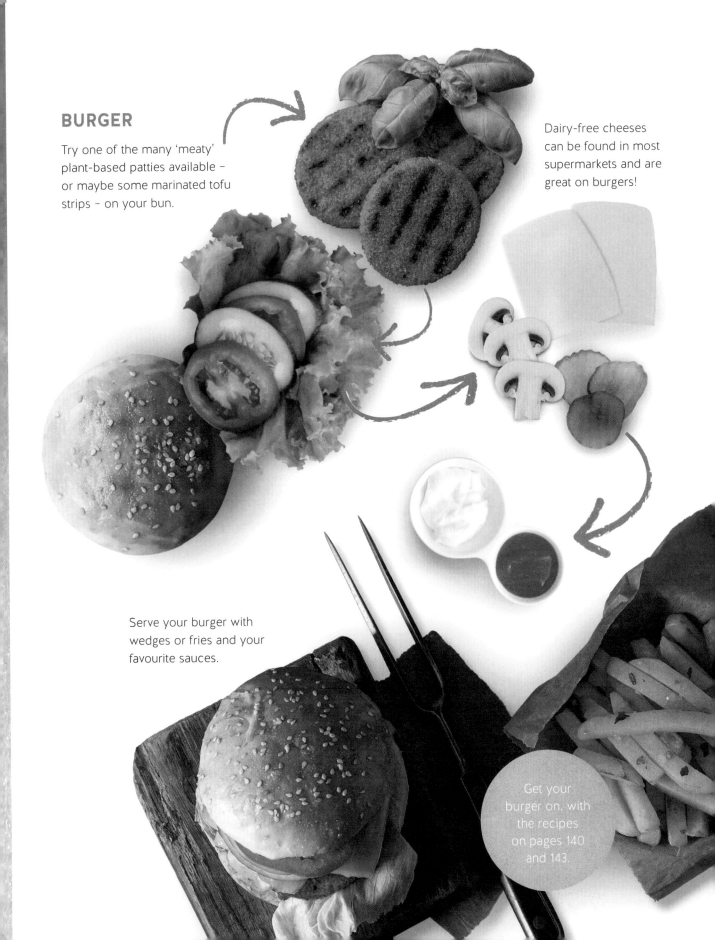

BURGER

Try one of the many 'meaty' plant-based patties available – or maybe some marinated tofu strips – on your bun.

Dairy-free cheeses can be found in most supermarkets and are great on burgers!

Serve your burger with wedges or fries and your favourite sauces.

Get your burger on, with the recipes on pages 140 and 143.

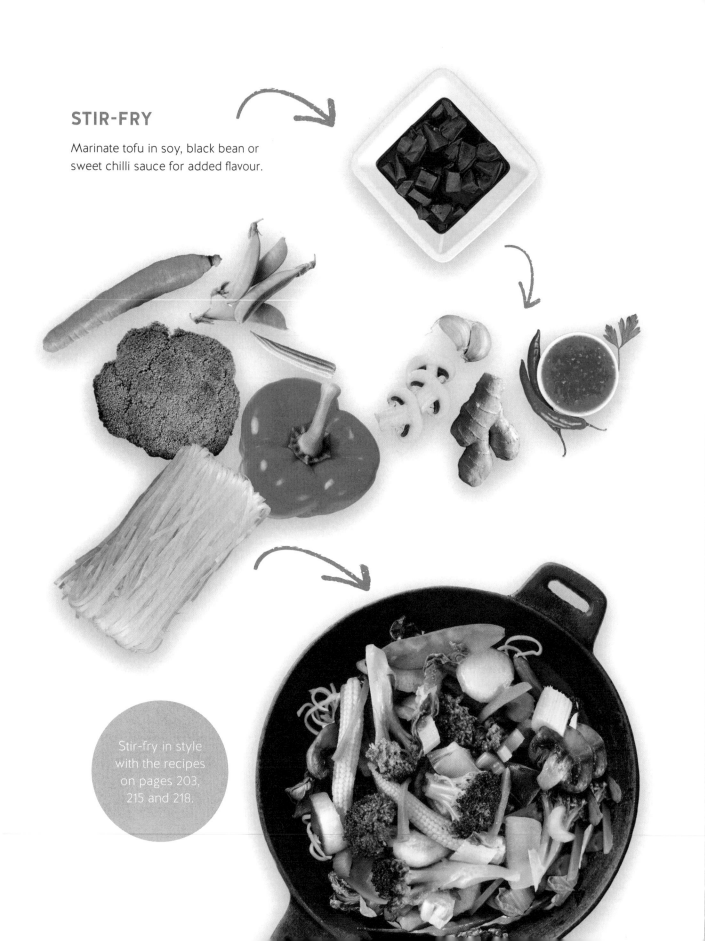

STIR-FRY

Marinate tofu in soy, black bean or sweet chilli sauce for added flavour.

Stir-fry in style with the recipes on pages 203, 215 and 218.

BURRITO

Throw in some cooked black beans or red kidney beans for your protein fix. Add salsa and dairy-free cheese for extra flavour.

Create great Mexican-inspired food with the recipes on pages 99, 185 and 172.

Can't see your favourite meal?

Plug a description into Google, add the word 'vegan' and away you go!

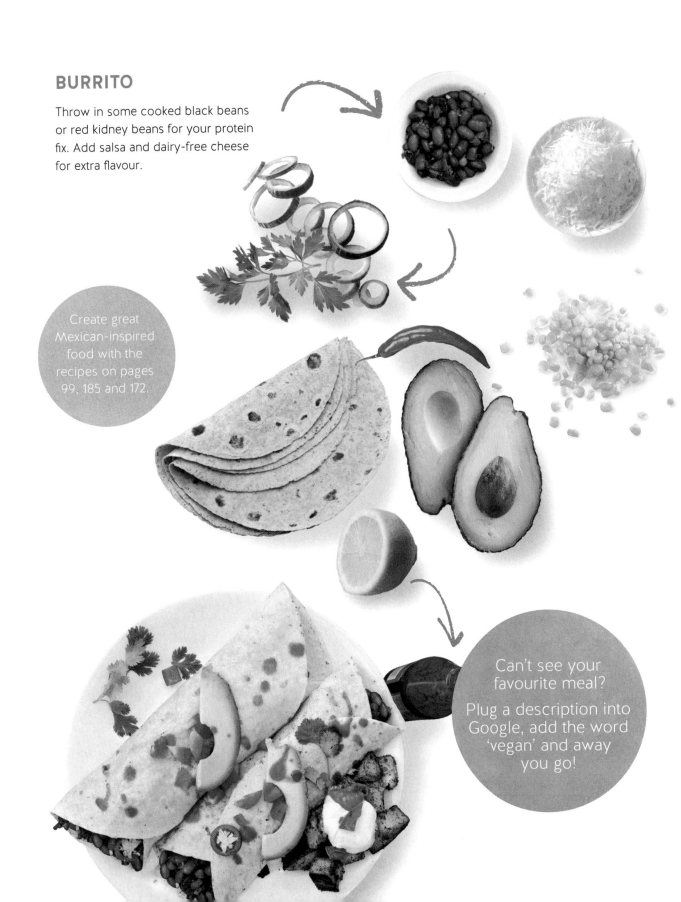

Your basic kitchen toolkit

You can whip up a meat-free storm in any old kitchen. But if you want to make your cooking fun and easy, having these items on hand will give you an edge.

HIGH-POWERED BLENDER To put it bluntly, a little $20 blender from the supermarket isn't going to cut it here. That said, there's no need to go crazy and mortgage the house to get a super-fancy one you see on late-night infomercials! While those monsters might be able to blend up a brick with just the flick of a switch, the most challenging things you'll face in this book are nuts and vegies. While a good blender can be a fairly sizeable investment, if you look after it, it'll last for years. Once you get in the groove of using it for everything from breakfast smoothies to soups, desserts and sauces, you can be sure you're getting your money's worth.

STICK BLENDER You could scrimp a little on this kitchen item – you don't need to get a top-of-the-line brand to do the trick. A stick blender makes pureeing soups and sauces an absolute dream.

THREE SHARP KNIVES A medium-sized good-quality chef's knife – or a Japanese santoku knife – will do pretty much everything you need in the kitchen. A little paring knife is handy for more delicate tasks like de-stemming mushrooms, getting the spiky bits out of pineapples or cutting cherry tomatoes into cute retro buffet shapes. We also highly recommend a good serrated bread knife. You might like to have more knives in your arsenal, but the only requirement is that you keep them all sharp. Because, truth be told, dull knives are responsible for more kitchen accidents than sharp ones. Sharp knives slice through even tough pumpkin skins with ease, without any of that frustrated sawing that can so easily result in a slip – and a trip to the ER.

VEGETABLE PEELER We know you can get these for $1 or so at the supermarket, but it's worth shelling out a few bucks for a heavier, more ergonomic model. You'll probably never have to buy one again, and your hand won't cramp after peeling a single potato.

CAST-IRON FRYPAN AND AN ENAMELLED FRENCH OVEN (OR THREE)

Enamelled French (or Dutch, we're not trying to start any wars here) ovens are perfect for cooking beans from scratch (see page 61), creating rich pasta sauces or slow simmering soups. Uncoated cast-iron frypans brown and crisp up tofu or potatoes like nobody's business. They do need a little love to keep in tip-top shape, but all that involves is hand washing them, drying thoroughly and coating with a little olive oil. Over time, you'll create a naturally non-stick patina – and a pan that is truly, uniquely yours.

BAMBOO CHOPPING BOARDS AND SPOONS These eco-friendly boards are not only kinder on your knives than glass or plastic, they're also perfect for pressing tofu (see our technique on page 60). Bamboo or wooden spoons are also an absolute must if you're using some of that lovely enamelled cast-iron cookware, because metal utensils will damage them.

ODDMENTS Measuring spoons, muffin and cake tins, a variety of mixing bowls, a couple of heavy roasting tins, a large ovenproof casserole dish or two and a range of different saucepans. Throw in some tongs, plastic spatulas, a potato masher, delicate sieve and heavy-duty colander, plus a wire rack for cooling, and you're all set!

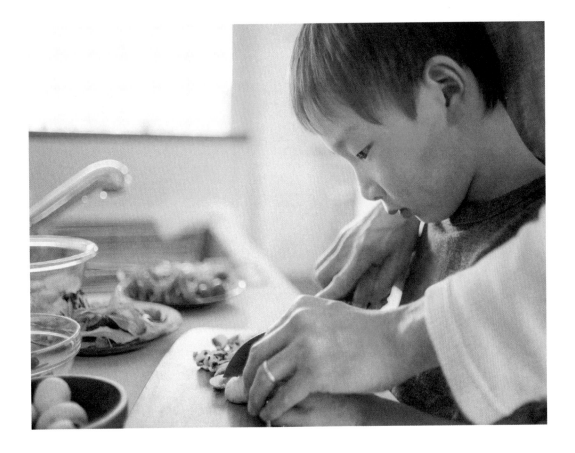

Ingredients

TOFU – THE SECRET ART TO MAKING IT GREAT!

When treated with a little care, tofu is not only delicious and nutritious, it's also the perfect animal-friendly solution to create mayo, quiches, cakes, breakfasts, barbecues – and everything in between. Here are a few simple tips to get you playing like an all-star in the tofu game:

1   **Find the right type.** Half the art of using tofu is picking the right type. 'Silken' and 'soft' styles of tofu have a wobbly jelly-like texture and are great for creamy and blended dishes such as sauces, dips, smoothies and desserts. 'Firm' and 'extra firm' are denser and hold their shape better. They will absorb flavour well (especially when pressed) and are great in stir-fries, marinated, baked, grilled or crumbled to make scrambled tofu (see page 70).

2   **Press it.** Removing excess moisture from your tofu can help ensure you don't water down your flavours – and pressed tofu will soak up marinades like a sponge. Simply wrap a block of firm tofu (don't try this with silken!) in a clean tea towel, then sandwich it between two chopping boards. Weigh it down with a cookbook or two and prop it up on an angle if you can, to help squeeze out the water. This should take only about 20–30 minutes.

3   **Drain it.** You shouldn't be rough with silken tofu. Usually, you won't need to expel any water as silken tofu's delicate texture is perfect in soups or baking. But when the occasion calls for it, gently place silken tofu in a colander or sieve lined with a clean tea towel and set over a plate or dish. Leave it to drip dry for at least 30 minutes.

4   **Freeze it.** Frozen and defrosted firm tofu goes through an almost magical metamorphosis, transforming into a chewier form that can withstand some rough-housing in stir-fries and it also goes great on the barbecue. Once defrosted, previously frozen tofu can be pressed to remove excess water by wrapping it in a clean tea towel and gently pressing it between your palms over the sink. Just don't squeeze too hard or it'll fall apart.

WTF (WHAT'S THAT FOOD)?

TOFU Made from soybeans, tofu comes in a variety of textures. It's high in protein, low in fat and a great addition to stir-fries, curries, wraps and so much more!

TEMPEH (TEM-PAY) Similar to tofu but with a 'meatier' texture, tempeh is perfect on a burger or when added to bulk up a salad.

NUTRITIONAL YEAST This nutty-flavoured condiment is delicious and a great source of B vitamins. Use it to make cheesy dairy-free sauces and in place of parmesan.

COOKING DRIED BEANS

Having a few tins of beans in the pantry is undoubtedly convenient, but cooking your own dried beans from scratch will not only save you a ton of money, but leftovers are also easily frozen for later use in a tasty and quick protein- and nutrient-rich midweek meal. So, if you're just pottering around the house on a lazy afternoon, why not cook up a pot of beans? Not only will you feel like a pioneering prairie homesteader, you'll also be qualified to wear a grin of smug self-satisfaction: yes, you are the kind of real grown-up, adult person who can plan ahead and boil your own beans.

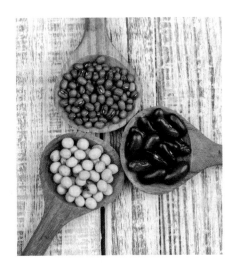

Three simple things to remember when cooking dried beans:

1   **Step away from the salt shaker.** NEVER add salt during cooking. While it's true that legumes love seasoning *after* they've been cooked, adding salt during cooking will slow down the process and can result in tough beans.

2   **Check the use-by date.** Although they do look like they might survive the apocalypse, dried beans are actually at their absolute best within one year. You can still use them after that time – just keep in mind that they will probably take longer to cook.

3   **Soak your heart out.** Always try to soak beans for a minimum of 8 hours, or preferably overnight, before cooking. Get in the habit of having a bowl soaking on your kitchen bench or in the fridge – it's easy to cook up a big batch and, remember, leftovers can be frozen.

Cooking dried beans couldn't be simpler. Soak beans overnight. Don't drain them, but instead place them with their soaking water – to preserve as many vitamins as possible – in a large saucepan or stockpot. Add enough water to cover the beans by at least 5 cm and bring to the boil. Skim off any foam that rises to the surface. Reduce the heat to low and simmer, uncovered, for anything between 30 minutes and 1 hour 30 minutes until the beans are tender – you should be able to squash one easily against the side of the pot – but not completely falling apart. Don't worry, you don't have to pay much attention during cooking. Simply stir occasionally to make sure the beans aren't sticking, and ensure the water doesn't dry up, adding more water if needed. If freezing or as required for a recipe, you may need to drain the beans at this stage. Otherwise, set aside until ready to add – liquid and all – to a soup, stew, casserole or chilli for maximum nutrition.

WARNING Never eat raw beans! Raw beans contain lectins – a protein that humans can't digest and which can make you ill. Kidney beans have particularly high concentrations. If you're soaking your own beans, these lectins are easily broken down by cooking. And if you're using tinned beans, these are pre-cooked.

THERE'S OIL – AND THEN THERE'S OIL

It's certainly more than possible to fill a whole pantry shelf (or three) just with different kinds of cooking oils, sauces and condiments. We're not judging – variety is the spice of life, after all. But, if you're short on space, these five oils will guide you wonderfully through most of the cooking adventures in this book.

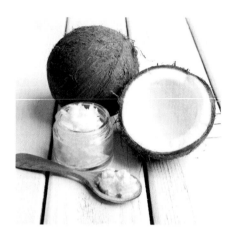

COCONUT OIL Solid creamy-white at room temperature, coconut oil melts easily into a clear liquid when warmed in the microwave or in a saucepan. With antibacterial properties and a high smoke point, coconut oil's rich and creamy flavour is perfect for frying, sautéing or roasting and it can be brushed on or poured over vegies before barbecuing. It can have quite a strong coconut aroma and taste, which makes it perfect for all Thai and Indian meals, but it also comes in a refined form with a very mild coconut flavour that is ideal for baking and sweet treats, or whenever you don't want strong coconut aromatics.

OLIVE OIL From antioxidant-rich strong extra virgin to subtle extra-light, olive oil is fantastic drizzled over cooked vegetables, whisked into salad dressings or simply served alongside fresh, crusty bread for dunking. The smoke point of extra virgin olive oil is approximately 200°C – be careful to not heat it over that temperature or you may spoil this delicate oil.

GRAPESEED OR RICE BRAN OIL Both have a high smoke point, making them good choices for shallow-, deep- or stir-frying. Their neutral taste is well suited for baking or in recipes when you don't want a coconut or olive flavour to come through.

FLAXSEED OIL Flaxseed oil (sometimes called linseed oil) is one of the best plant sources of Omega-3 fatty acids. These healthy fats can help lower blood pressure, cholesterol levels and inflammation. Not a cooking oil, flaxseed oil doesn't cope well with heat. It's best stored in the fridge and added to dishes after cooking. While flaxseed oil is full of health benefits, some people find its crisp, nutty flavour takes some getting used to. If you find the taste to be too dominant, try mixing it with olive oil or other flavoursome ingredients such as garlic or lemon juice in salad dressings.

SESAME OIL Cold-pressed sesame oil is best refrigerated, as like flaxseed oil it is sensitive to heat. High in healthy fats, this pale oil is lovely in salad dressings. Toasted golden sesame oil is your secret ingredient to make everything delicious! With its rich nutty flavour, toasted sesame oil is particularly great in salads and Asian cooking. Adding just a few drops towards the end of cooking fried rice, noodles, stir-fries, dressings or dipping sauces will transform your meal into restaurant-quality food in seconds.

COW-FRIENDLY CREAMINESS

From potato bakes to scones, laksa to stroganoff, there are plenty of ways to dollop a big spoonful of creaminess into your favourite dishes. Coconut cream imparts a touch of luxury to stir-fries and curries. Silken tofu is a perfect filler for quiches (see page 105) and mayo (see page 157).

Blended cashews are the go-to for decadent pastas and sauces (see pages 131, 159, 181 and 185, to name just a few). Simply soak raw cashews overnight in a sealed container in the fridge, blitz up in your blender the next day and *voila!* You've got yourself some cow-approved cream that we guarantee your guests will approve of, too.

It's an emergency! Unexpected guests arrive and you need a creamy pasta bake bubbling and on the table in an hour? Don't stress. Pour boiling water over your raw cashews and leave them to soak for at least 15 minutes before pouring into a blender and pulsing until smooth. The results won't be as silky as cashews soaked overnight, but they'll still be fine.

EGG-FREE BAKING

Cookies, muffins, cakes? No egg? No problem. When baking, in the place of one egg, try these healthy options. Depending on the recipe, some work better than others, so feel free to experiment.

Commercial egg replacer (such as No Egg)

½ mashed banana

1 tablespoon vinegar + 1 teaspoon bicarbonate of soda

½ cup apple sauce

¼ cup silken tofu

1 tablespoon ground flaxseed + 3 tablespoons water

¼ cup soy yoghurt

MAGIC MERINGUES

This may sound crazy ... but the liquid in a tin of chickpeas has seemingly supernatural powers. Sometimes called 'aquafaba', you can whip it up like egg whites and make amazing meringues, pavlovas, macarons and more! See page 240 for our amazing meringue recipe.

Part Three

111 Delicious
Recipes
for Life

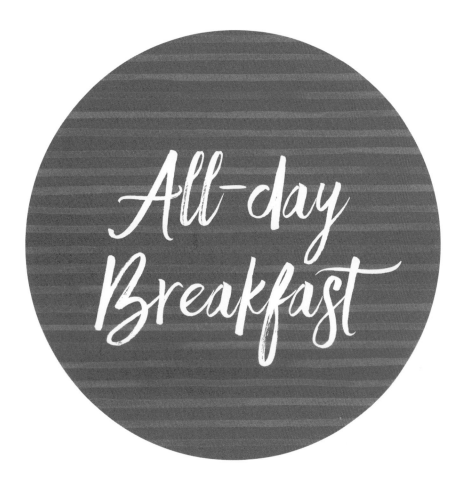

All-day Breakfast

Whether you like muesli, smoothies or a stack of fluffy pancakes drenched with syrup, start your day the compassionate way with our breakfasts for champions! (And if you feel like French toast at midnight, slip down to the kitchen in your robe and dig in. We won't tell.)

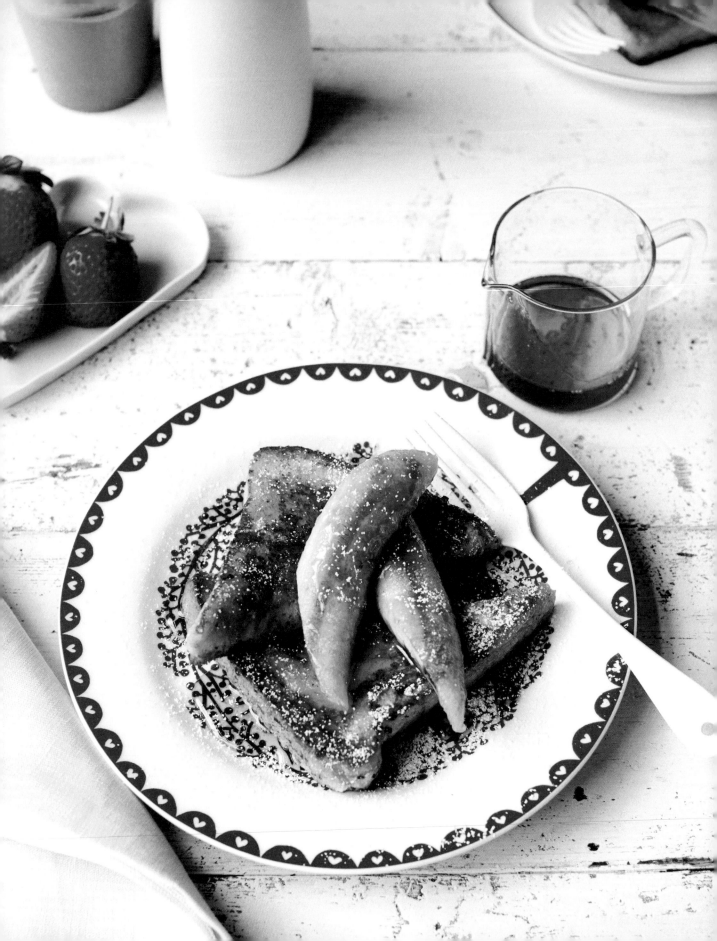

French Toast

SERVES 4

*Sweet, custardy, crunchy ... and a brilliant way to use up a slightly stale loaf. It's best
to use a nice dense bread for this – a light rye or sourdough works particularly well.
Make sure your slices are lovely and thick, to soak up all the spiced milk.*

8 thick slices of bread
1 cup soy milk, or any dairy-free milk
2–3 teaspoons brown sugar
½ teaspoon ground cinnamon
a pinch of ground nutmeg
2 teaspoons pure vanilla extract
1 tablespoon cornflour
1 tablespoon self-raising flour
a pinch of salt
2 tablespoons neutral-tasting oil,
   such as rice bran, for pan-frying
maple syrup, to serve
fresh berries or sliced banana,
   to serve
sifted icing sugar, for dusting

- If your bread is fresh, give it a quick turn in the toaster, to stop it falling apart when you dip it in the milk mixture.
- Meanwhile, whisk together the soy milk, sugar, cinnamon, nutmeg, vanilla, cornflour, flour and salt, then pour into a wide, shallow bowl for ease of dipping.
- Melt the oil in a non-stick frying pan over medium–high heat.
- Dunk both sides of a few slices of bread in the milk mixture, then transfer to the hot pan. Cook for a few minutes, until the underside is nicely browned, then carefully flip the slices over and brown the other side. Remove from the pan and cook the remaining slices in the same way.
- Serve immediately, with maple syrup, fresh berries or sliced banana on the side, and a dusting of icing sugar.

Variations

- Try coconut milk for a tropical flavour, and top with cubed mango and a sprinkling of coconut flakes.
- Use chickpea flour (besan) instead of plain flour, for a more savoury flavour that works a treat with Smoky tempeh strips (page 85) and maple syrup.

Tip

For a special treat,
sauté banana slices in
1 tablespoon coconut oil and
1–2 teaspoons brown sugar.
When starting to caramelise,
add a tablespoon of rum and
cook for a few seconds.
Serve with a sprinkling of
ground cinnamon.

Spinach and Tofu Scramble

SERVES 2

After just one taste, this easy, filling and flavoursome breakfast may well become a weekend staple at your house. We recommend serving it on toasted Turkish bread with fresh avocado and a slice of lemon. Once you've perfected this version, experiment with other flavours.

1 tablespoon olive oil
1 onion, diced
1 garlic clove, crushed
250 g medium-firm tofu
½ cup vegan chicken-style stock
1 teaspoon ground turmeric
2 teaspoons soy sauce
100 g baby spinach leaves
¼ lemon, to squeeze

- Heat the olive oil in a frying pan over high heat. Add the onion and a pinch of salt and stir for about 1 minute, or until soft. (The salt will help stop the onion sticking to the pan.) Add the garlic and stir for another 30 seconds, or until fragrant.

- Crumble the tofu into the pan with your hands; keeping some chunks bigger is fine. Stir to combine, then cook for 2–3 minutes, gradually adding the stock to keep the scramble moist. You may not need all the stock, but some excess liquid in the pan is okay as it will reduce as it continues cooking.

- Add the turmeric, soy sauce and spinach. Stir until the tofu is coated, the spinach is soft, and any excess stock has reduced.

- Finish with a squeeze of lemon juice and serve immediately.

Variations

- Instead of seasoning with turmeric, soy sauce and spinach, try one of these variations:

- For a mushroom and pesto scramble, add 1 cup quartered mushrooms and a handful of chopped sundried tomatoes to the tofu and cook until the mushrooms are soft. Just before serving, stir through 1–2 tablespoons of fresh basil pesto, from the Pesto pasta bake recipe on page 190).

- For a fresh avocado salsa scramble, combine 1 diced avocado and 8–10 halved cherry tomatoes in a bowl. Season with lemon juice, salt and chopped mint. When cooking the tofu, add 2 tablespoons nutritional yeast and a handful of chopped fresh chives. Serve topped with the avocado and tomato salsa.

Tip
To make this recipe gluten-free, swap the soy sauce for gluten-free tamari.

Bircher Muesli

SERVES 4

This 'summer porridge' is full of slow-release energy to help you power through your day. Prepare most of it the night before, and it'll come together in minutes. You can use any combination of fruits and nuts – try this version as a guide, then follow your tastebuds.

2 cups rolled oats

2–3 tablespoons mixed seeds (such as chia, flaxseed, sunflower, pumpkin and sesame)

2–3 tablespoons maple syrup or agave syrup, plus extra to serve

1 teaspoon pure vanilla extract

1 teaspoon ground cinnamon

2 apples, cored and grated

a handful of frozen blueberries (or mixed berries)

1 cup fresh orange juice

1 cup dairy-free milk, plus extra to serve

coconut yoghurt, to serve

fresh fruits, to serve

flaked almonds, chopped walnuts or pecans, to serve

- Combine the oats, mixed seeds, maple syrup, vanilla, cinnamon, grated apple and frozen blueberries in a large bowl. Pour in the orange juice and dairy-free milk and stir well to combine. Cover and leave overnight in the fridge.

- The next morning, fold through about a tablespoon of coconut yoghurt, and enough dairy-free milk to reach your desired consistency. (As with porridge, this is a very personal thing: some love their bircher muesli firm, others spoonable, so let everyone adjust their own to avoid breakfast skirmishes.)

- Spoon into serving bowls and top with extra coconut yoghurt, fresh fruits and flaked almonds or chopped nuts.

- Serve extra maple syrup or agave syrup on the side for those with a super sweet tooth.

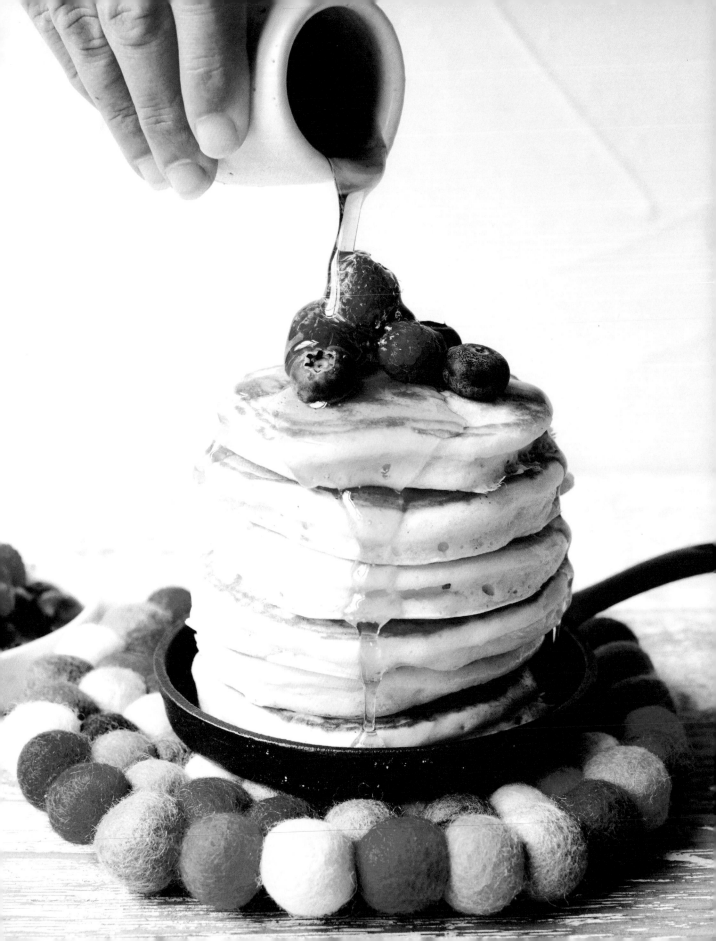

Pancakes

SERVES 2-3

This no-egg, no-fuss recipe is quick and easy. Serve these fluffy pancakes with maple syrup, lemon and a sprinkling of sugar – or for a fancy brunch dish to impress your in-laws, go all out with caramelised banana, brown sugar and rum (see tip page 69).

2 tablespoons vegetable oil, plus extra for pan-frying
1 cup plain flour
2 tablespoons sugar
1 tablespoon baking powder
1 teaspoon cornflour
1⅓ cups soy milk, or other dairy-free milk, adjust to suit your preference
1 teaspoon pure vanilla extract

• Lightly oil a non-stick frying pan and place over medium–low heat. If you don't have a non-stick frying pan, use some dairy-free margarine to cook the pancakes, along with a little oil.

• Combine the flour, sugar, baking powder and cornflour in a mixing bowl. Add a pinch of salt. Gradually whisk in the soy milk, vanilla and the 2 tablespoons vegetable oil until smooth. If you like your pancakes thinner or thicker, add a little more or a little less soy milk.

• Pour about ¼–⅓ cup of pancake batter into the pan. The pancake should start bubbling; flip it over when it's firm enough to do so. (If you're feeling brave, flip it straight out of the pan and back in again – although it's probably best to practise this first before trying it in front of company!)

• Cook and flip again, if needed, until golden on both sides. Remove from the pan and keep warm while cooking the remaining pancake batter. You should end up with 6–8 pancakes.

• Serve warm, with your choice of toppings.

Tip

The right heat can make all the difference. If your pancakes aren't bubbling, try turning the heat up slightly; if they are burning, turn the heat down.

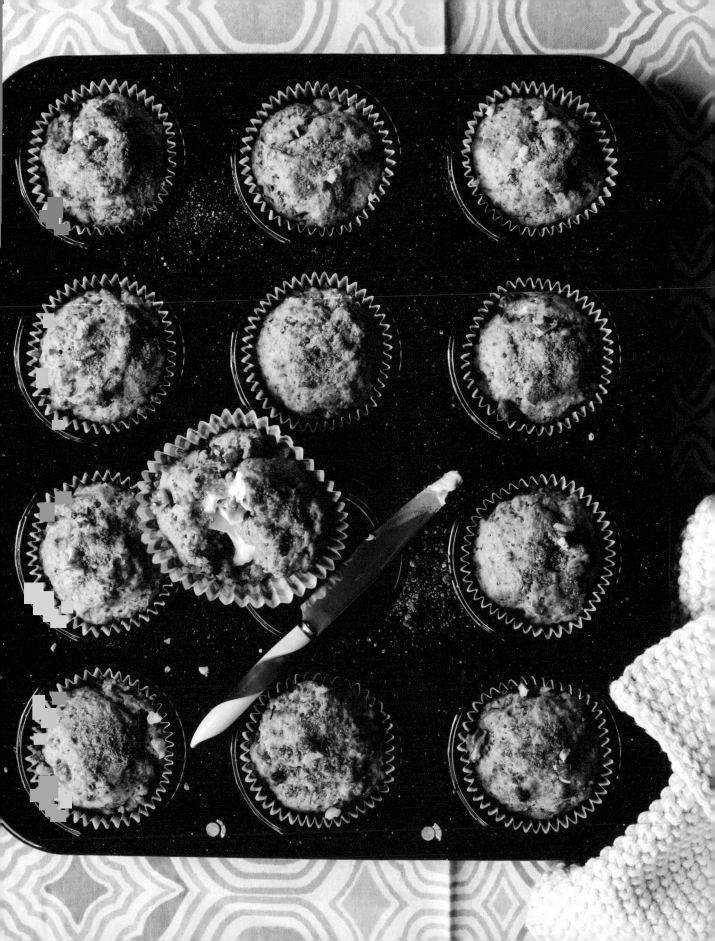

Nutty Banana–Date Breakfast Muffins

MAKES 12 MUFFINS

There's no need to feel guilty about eating 'cake' for breakfast with these wholesome muffins, filled with Omega-rich flaxseed goodness. Don't let the thought of wholemeal flour deter you – all you'll taste is a nutty undertone that complements the walnuts.

1½ cups soy milk

¼ cup ground flaxseeds

2 ripe bananas, mashed

zest and juice of 1 lemon

1 cup plain flour

¾ cup self-raising wholemeal flour

2 teaspoons baking powder

1 teaspoon ground cinnamon

½ teaspoon mixed spice

a pinch of salt

½ cup pitted dates, roughly chopped

½ cup walnuts, chopped

¼ cup mild-flavoured olive oil
   or rice bran oil

½ cup brown sugar, to taste

2 teaspoons pure vanilla extract

raw sugar, for sprinkling

- Preheat the oven to 200°C conventional, or 180°C fan-forced. Line a 12-hole muffin tin with non-stick paper cases.

- In a small bowl, mix together the soy milk, flaxseeds, banana, lemon zest and lemon juice. Set aside until the mixture has thickened slightly.

- Meanwhile, into a large bowl, sift together the flours, baking powder, cinnamon, mixed spice and salt. Stir well, then add the chopped dates and walnuts, and give another quick mix.

- Add the olive oil to the lemony flaxseed milk, along with the brown sugar and vanilla. Whisk until combined.

- Make a well in the dry ingredients. Pour in the milk mixture and stir until just combined, but don't be too fussy – some dry patches are perfectly fine. Be careful not to overmix or you'll end up with tough muffins!

- Quickly spoon the mixture into the muffin cases, then sprinkle with the raw sugar (it will create a nice crunchy top).

- Bake for about 20–25 minutes, or until the muffins are golden brown; if a skewer inserted into the centre of a muffin comes out clean, you're done! If not, bake for another 2–5 minutes. (If you accidentally overcook them, don't stress: a quick zap in the microwave later will soften them up.)

- Transfer to a cooling rack and leave to sit for 5 minutes, before turning out of the tin. These little babies are best eaten warm.

Variations

- Instead of bananas and walnuts, use blackberries, blueberries, raspberries or mixed berries, and a combination of orange and lemon zest.

- To make apple and cinnamon muffins, replace the banana with diced Granny Smith apples, and add a pinch more cinnamon.

- Feel like 'fruit toast' muffins? Instead of the dates and walnuts, use 1½ cups mixed dried sultanas, raisins, currants and mixed peel.

Ultimate TLTs with Avocado

SERVES 2

An animal-friendly take on the traditional BLT breakfast roll, this mouthwatering TLT (tofu, lettuce and tomato) is sure to become a regular feature of your brunch repertoire. The crispy smoky-maple tofu is wonderful with the creaminess of fresh avocado, delivering a burst of flavour with every bite. The tofu is best if left to marinate overnight, but we've got you covered with a quick shortcut if you wake up one morning hankering for a TLT.

⅓ cup soy sauce

⅓ cup maple syrup

2 teaspoons liquid smoke

200 g firm tofu, sliced into thin rectangular strips

1 tablespoon rice bran or grapeseed oil, for pan-frying

1 ripe avocado

2 teaspoons fresh lemon juice

¼ teaspoon salt

2 Turkish bread rolls, split open

2 tablespoons egg-free mayonnaise

1 ripe tomato, sliced

4 cos lettuce leaves

- In a bowl or airtight container, combine the soy sauce, maple syrup, liquid smoke and ½ cup water. Submerge the tofu strips in the marinade, then cover and refrigerate for at least 2 hours, or overnight if possible.

- Heat the oil in a frying pan over high heat. Add the tofu strips, along with 2–3 tablespoons of the marinade. Cook for 2–3 minutes, then flip the strips over and cook until the marinade has been absorbed, and the tofu is browned and crispy on both sides.

- Meanwhile, mash the avocado in a bowl with the lemon juice and salt.

- To assemble your epic TLTs, open out the Turkish rolls, smear them with the avocado spread, then add the crispy tofu strips, and mayonnaise to taste. Top the whole thing off with some juicy tomato slices and lettuce leaves, then carry those rolls to the table like the champion you are.

Tip

If you don't have time to marinate the tofu for 2 hours, simply add more of the marinade to the pan when cooking the tofu.

Avocado Delight on Sourdough

SERVES 1

~~~~~~~~~~

Here's one to excite avocado lovers. Just when you thought nothing could get better than fresh, creamy avocado on toast, the added zest, crunch and pops of fruitiness in this healthy breakfast or snack are, well, simply delightful.

1 teaspoon raw almonds
1 avocado
1 mint leaf, sliced or chopped
3 small slices of ruby-red grapefruit
1 tablespoon lemon juice
1 tablespoon olive oil
2 slices of sourdough bread
a pinch of Himalayan rock salt
a pinch of black pepper
4 thin slices of red radish
½ teaspoon pepitas
½ teaspoon sunflower seeds

- Crush the almonds using a mortar and pestle or food processor. Don't crush them too fine; keep them nice and coarse. Place in a bowl.

- Cut the avocado in half and remove the stone. Dice the flesh and add to the almonds with the mint, grapefruit, lemon juice and olive oil. Toss gently but thoroughly.

- Toast the bread and place on a plate. Top with the avocado mix, and a sprinkling of rock salt and black pepper. Garnish with the radish, sprinkle with the seeds and enjoy right away.

Recipe contributed by 'What You Eat' Café

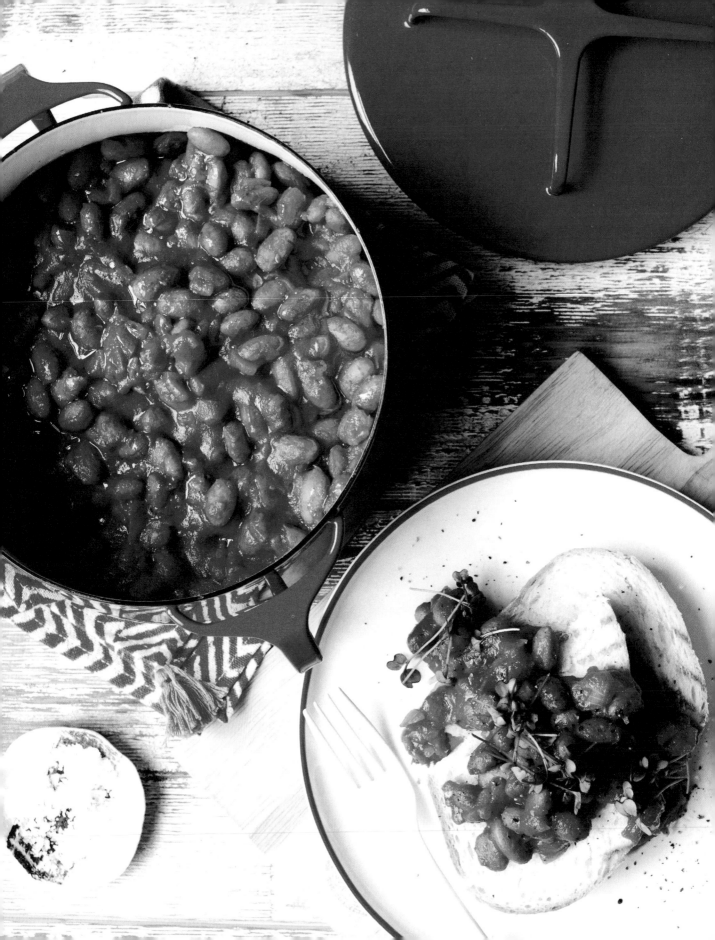

Homestyle Baked Beans

SERVES 4, OR 2, WITH PLENTY OF FREEZABLE LEFTOVERS

You'll never go back to regular baked beans after trying these! The spices and maple syrup work together beautifully to create a rich, smoky take on an old favourite. Serve on toast with avocado slices – or as part of a full brunch spread with Smoky tempeh strips (page 85) and the Seeded potato rösti (page 87).

1–2 tablespoons olive oil

1 small onion, finely diced

2 garlic cloves, crushed

½ teaspoon salt

¼ teaspoon ground allspice

1 tablespoon vegan Worcestershire sauce

1 tablespoon agave syrup or maple syrup

350 ml tomato passata

1 bay leaf

2 teaspoons liquid smoke (see tip), or smoked paprika (optional)

1–1½ cups vegetable stock or water

4 cups cooked borlotti or cannellini beans; tinned beans are fine

toasted bread and microherbs (optional), to serve

- Preheat the oven to 200°C conventional, or 180°C fan-forced.

- Heat the olive oil in a large frying pan. Add the onion and fry, stirring regularly, over medium–high heat for 10 minutes, or until translucent.

- Add the garlic and fry, stirring constantly, for another minute. Stir in the salt, allspice, Worcestershire sauce, agave syrup and passata. Add the bay leaf and the liquid smoke, if using. Stir in enough stock to reach your desired consistency; you may not need it all. Bring to the boil, then reduce the heat and simmer for 5 minutes.

- Gently stir the cooked beans through the sauce mixture, then pour the whole lot into a large baking dish. Cover with the lid or foil, then transfer to the oven and bake for 20 minutes, stirring carefully halfway through cooking. If you'd like a thicker sauce, cook for a further 10 minutes with the lid off; if you like it saucier, gently stir in a little boiling water.

- Remove from the oven and allow to stand for 10 minutes. Discard the bay leaf before serving.

Variations

- For barbecue-flavoured baked beans, replace the liquid smoke, Worcestershire sauce and agave syrup with ¼ cup of your favourite barbecue sauce.

- For spicy baked beans, replace the liquid smoke with your favourite chilli sauce. You could also add 1 teaspoon ground cumin, and substitute half the beans with cooked red kidney beans for an Old West chilli flavour.

- Roughly chopped coriander makes a tasty garnish.

Tip

Liquid smoke is available in health food stores and some supermarkets and adds a smoky flavour to dishes.

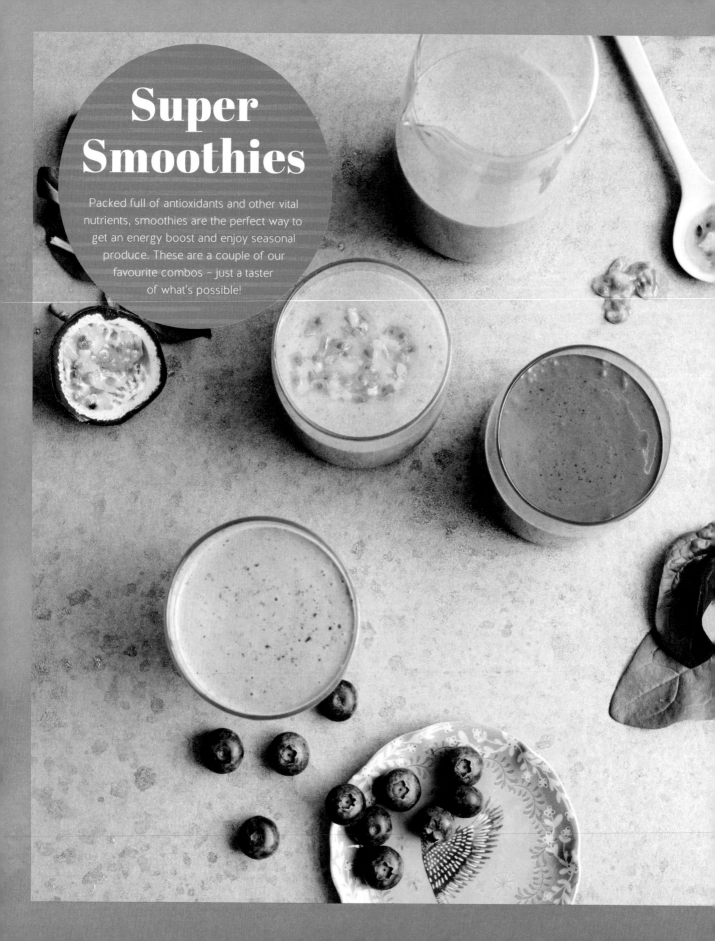

Super Smoothies

Packed full of antioxidants and other vital nutrients, smoothies are the perfect way to get an energy boost and enjoy seasonal produce. These are a couple of our favourite combos – just a taster of what's possible!

Passion for Greens

SERVES 2

With nutrient-rich spinach, sweet banana, fragrant passionfruit and refreshing coconut water, this smoothie is packed full of goodness. For an extra immunity boost, add some fresh ginger, kale or matcha powder.

a large handful of baby spinach leaves
2–3 ripe bananas, peeled
½ cucumber
1 cup coconut water
4–8 ice cubes
pulp of 3 passionfruit

- Beginning with the baby spinach leaves, add all the ingredients to a blender – except the passionfruit pulp. Process until smooth, then pour into two glasses. Spoon the passionfruit pulp over the top and serve.

Variation: If you can't get fresh passionfruit, or would like a super-smooth drink, use peeled fresh or frozen mango chunks instead.

Blueberry Banana Bliss

SERVES 2

Perfectly purple, with a hint of vanilla and cinnamon spice, this smoothie is bursting with antioxidants.

1 cup frozen blueberries (see variation)
2 frozen ripe bananas, chopped
1 cup soy milk
½ cup coconut milk
1 teaspoon pure vanilla extract
1 teaspoon ground cinnamon

- Add all the ingredients to a blender and process until smooth. If using fresh blueberries or unfrozen banana, add a handful of ice.
- Pour into two glasses and serve.

Variation: For a mixed berry smoothie, add ½ cup raspberries or strawberries, or both!

Choc Protein Punch

SERVES 2

For a healthy way to start the day, or to replenish yourself after a workout, this delicious smoothie offers a stack of protein in one easy go. Add some flaxseed meal for an extra health hit.

1 cup soy milk
2 tablespoons chocolate-flavoured
    pea or rice protein powder (see tip)
½ cup frozen blueberries, strawberries
    or raspberries
1 heaped tablespoon natural
    peanut butter
1 ripe banana, peeled
1 teaspoon ground cinnamon

- Add all the ingredients to a blender. Process until smooth, pour into two glasses and serve.

Tip: If you're using a non-chocolate protein powder, simply add 1 teaspoon cocoa or cacao powder to achieve that delicious chocolatey taste.

White Beans with Rosemary

SERVES 4 AS A SIDE

The list of ingredients may be short, but they add up to a delicious protein-rich smash. These beans are perfect as a side with Seeded potato rösti (page 87) and avocado, or try them spooned on top of thick-cut garlic toast with a drizzle of extra virgin olive oil and a few slices of perfectly ripe tomato.

2 teaspoons olive oil

1 garlic clove, sliced

1 tablespoon finely chopped rosemary

1 thyme sprig

2 x 400 g tins cannellini beans, drained but not rinsed

1–1½ cups vegetable stock (depending on desired consistency)

1 bay leaf

extra virgin olive oil, for drizzling

chopped herbs such as thyme or parsley, to serve

garlic toast (see tip), to serve (optional)

- In a saucepan, gently heat the olive oil and garlic over low heat, along with a tiny pinch of salt to stop the garlic browning. After about 1 minute, once the oil is infused with garlic flavour, remove and discard the garlic. Add the chopped rosemary and thyme sprig and stir for 30 seconds, or until fragrant.

- Add 1½ tins of the cannellini beans. Stir to coat the beans with the herb-infused oil, then pour in enough stock to just cover the beans. Add the bay leaf.

- Increase the heat to medium, cover the pan and bring to a gentle simmer. Cook for about 5 minutes, then remove the bay leaf.

- Using a potato masher or fork, smash the beans into a rough paste. Add more stock now, if desired, some black pepper to taste, and the remaining whole cannellini beans. Stir gently to mix, trying to keep some beans whole for texture, until warmed through. Season to taste with salt and pepper.

- Spoon the beans into a serving dish. Drizzle with extra virgin olive oil, sprinkle with herbs and serve hot, with hot garlic toast if desired.

Tip

Toast thick slices of your favourite bread. While it's still hot, cut an unpeeled garlic clove in half and gently rub it over the toast to infuse it with garlic flavour. Sprinkle with salt and drizzle with olive oil, if desired. Serve hot.

Cacao and Goji Berry Granola

SERVES 6-8

*Packed with tasty superfoods, this crunchy granola will keep you energised all day.
The combination of caramelised syrup on toasty oats, seeds and nuts makes this
filling breakfast or snack so delicious that you'll forget it's good for you too!*

100 ml maple syrup

3 tablespoons coconut oil

3 tablespoons nut butter

½ cup raw cacao powder

1½ tablespoons ground cinnamon

3 teaspoons pure vanilla extract

4½ cups rolled oats

1½ cups raw almonds, chopped

¾ cup raw pepitas

¾ cup raw unsalted sunflower seeds

⅓ cup unsweetened flaked or
   shredded coconut

agave syrup or extra maple syrup,
   for drizzling

½ cup dried goji berries

⅓ cup chia seeds

¼ cup raw cacao nibs

- Preheat the oven to 150°C conventional, or 130°C fan-forced. Line two baking trays with baking paper.

- In a saucepan, mix the maple syrup, coconut oil and nut butter over medium heat. Add the cacao powder and cinnamon and bring to the boil. Reduce the heat and simmer for 5 minutes. Once it has reached a sticky consistency, stir in the vanilla and set aside.

- Meanwhile, in a large bowl, mix together the oats, almonds, pepitas, sunflower seeds and coconut.

- While the chocolate mixture is still warm, pour it over the oat mixture and mix well until everything is evenly coated.

- Spread the chocolate granola onto the two lined baking trays. Drizzle with agave or maple syrup to your desired level of sweetness. Wearing food-handling gloves, clump the granola together as best you can with your hands to create chunks. (Maple syrup won't clump the mixture together as much as agave syrup, but will still taste delicious.)

- Bake in the oven for 20–25 minutes, stirring every 10 minutes, and swapping the trays around in the oven so the granola cooks evenly.

- When the chocolate granola is golden brown, remove it from the oven; it should be slightly crispy, but not dry. Set it aside to cool for about 30 minutes, to harden into the texture of granola; during this time, resist the temptation to cover it or place it in a container.

- When the granola has completely cooled down, stir in the goji berries, chia seeds and cacao nibs.

- At this stage, you can store the granola in an airtight container at room temperature.

- Serve with seasonal fruit, extra goji berries and dairy-free milk.

- The granola is also delicious as a healthy snack when you're sprawled on the couch binge-watching your favourite series on telly!

Recipe contributed by 'What You Eat' Café

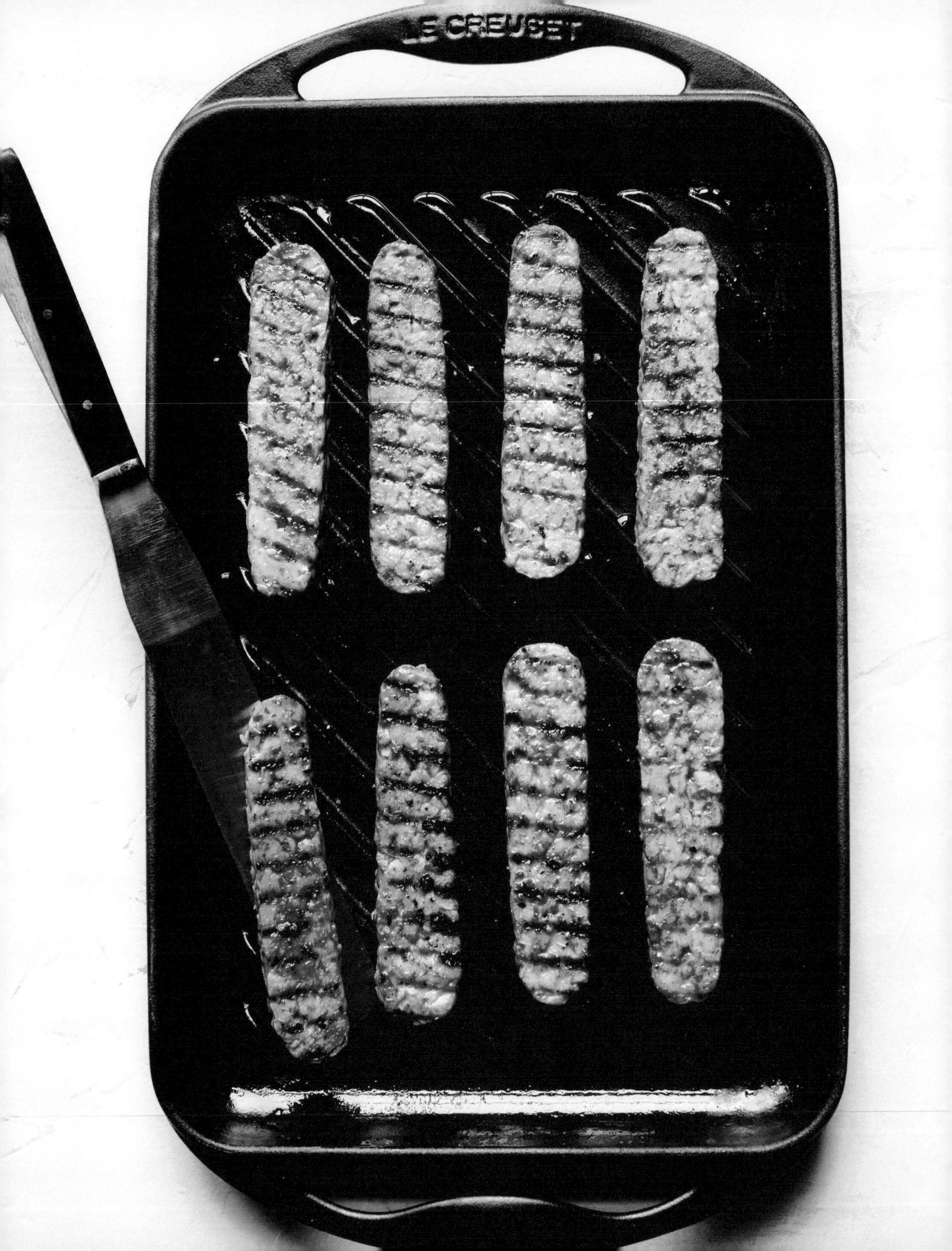
LE CREUSET

Smoky Tempeh Strips

SERVES 2-4

Crispy, salty, moreish and heart healthy, tempeh is a traditional Indonesian food that is rich in protein, fibre and vitamins. It's also a perfect base for many dishes as it soaks up marinades beautifully. Try these smoky strips as a breakfast side, crumbled atop a basic tomato pasta, crammed into a burrito or stuffed into an Ultimate TLT (page 76).

400 g packet tempeh, rinsed
  and drained
1 teaspoon smoked paprika (see tip)
1 teaspoon brown sugar
¼ cup soy sauce or tamari
3 garlic cloves, crushed
1 tablespoon olive oil
1 tablespoon apple cider vinegar
rice bran oil, for pan-frying

- Slice the tempeh lengthways into thin strips, then pack into a sandwich bag or airtight container.
- In a small bowl, whisk together the paprika, sugar, soy sauce, garlic, olive oil and vinegar, then pour over the tempeh. Toss the tempeh slices around until nicely coated.
- Seal and leave to marinate in the fridge for at least 1 hour, or overnight if possible, for maximum flavour.
- When you're ready to serve, heat a few tablespoons of rice bran oil in a frying pan over medium-high heat, then fry the tempeh slices until well browned. They're now ready to enjoy straight out of the pan, or to star in other recipes.

Variation

- For a more Italian-style flavour, dice the tempeh instead of slicing it, then replace the smoked paprika with 1 teaspoon ground fennel, 1 teaspoon chilli flakes and a pinch of ground dried sage. Fry until golden brown, then add to a tomato and baby spinach pasta sauce.

Tip

Liquid smoke can be used instead of the smoked paprika. It has a strong flavour, so start by adding just a couple of drops, and increase the amount to suit your taste.

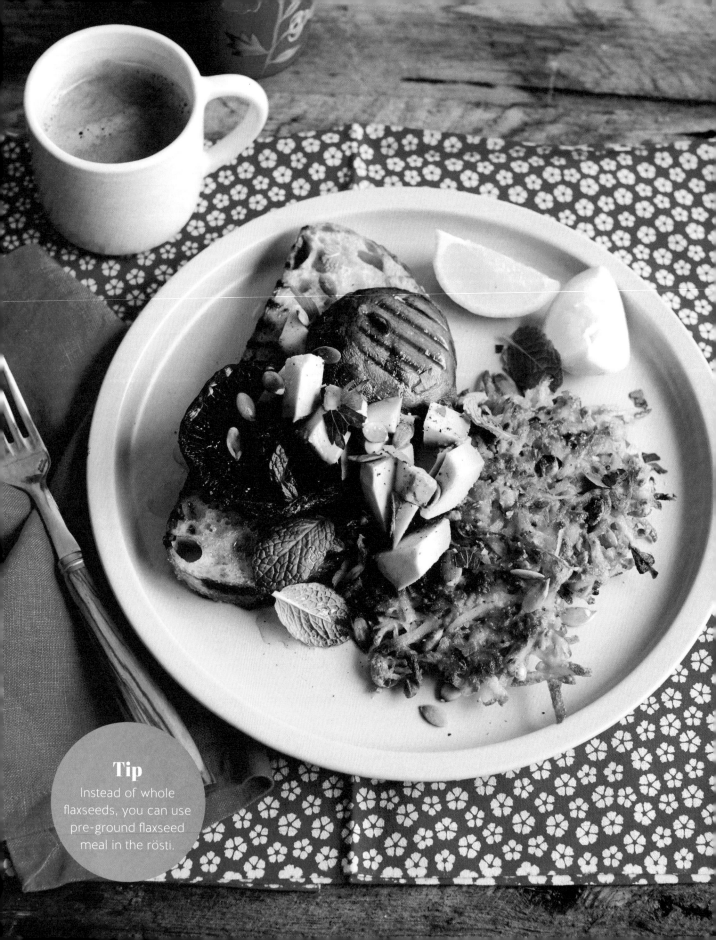

Tip
Instead of whole flaxseeds, you can use pre-ground flaxseed meal in the rösti.

Seeded Potato Rösti with Portobello Mushrooms and Avocado

SERVES 2-3

For breakfast or brunch, this tasty café-style dish goes down a treat. Crispy, crunchy potato rösti contrasts beautifully with creamy avocado; savoury mushrooms bring it all together. Add a sprig of fresh mint and we guarantee you'll enjoy every last bite.

If you're breakfasting with avocado lovers, you could even use a whole avocado here. The rösti is even more delicious topped with Rosemary and garlic marinated almond feta from (page 187)!

2-3 large or 4-6 small portobello mushrooms (1 or 2 per serve, depending on size)
½ avocado, diced
½ teaspoon olive oil
juice of ½ lemon
toasted sourdough bread slices, to serve
pepitas, for sprinkling
mint or parsley sprigs, to garnish

SEEDED POTATO RÖSTI

1½ tablespoons whole flaxseeds (see tip)
2 potatoes, peeled and grated
1½ tablespoons plain flour
1 tablespoon pepitas, chopped
1 tablespoon sunflower seeds, chopped
olive oil, for pan-frying

- To make the rösti, place the flaxseeds in a food processor and grind into a powder. Tip into a small bowl. Stir in 2 tablespoons water, mix well, then set aside for 10 minutes, or until the mixture forms a gel.

- Place the grated potato on a clean tea towel or paper towel, then press and squeeze out as much moisture as possible.

- Place the potato in a large bowl. Add the flour and flaxseed gel. Mix well, then add the pepitas and sunflower seeds and season with a pinch of salt and pepper.

- Pour a good amount of olive oil into a hot frying pan. Divide the rösti mixture into six small portions and use a fork to flatten and form each one into a circle about 1 cm thick and 8 cm wide; you may need to cook them in two batches, to avoid overcrowding the pan. Cook over medium heat for 8-10 minutes on each side, until golden and crispy.

- Meanwhile, in a separate frying pan, cook the mushrooms over medium heat for about 8 minutes on each side, until lightly browned, using a little olive oil if desired. Season to taste with salt and pepper.

- Just before serving, place the avocado in a bowl, drizzle with the olive oil and lemon juice, and sprinkle with salt.

- Arrange the warm rösti, mushrooms and sourdough toast on plates. Top with the avocado, sprinkle with pepitas, garnish with mint and serve straight away.

Recipe contributed by 'What You Eat' Café

Baked Berry Breakfast Oats

SERVES 4-6

These lightly spiced oats are studded with seasonal fruits, offering all the comfort and nutrition of a traditional, creamy porridge – without having to stand there stirring over a hot stove. This is a great dish for a lazy brunch with friends, and makes enough for Goldilocks and the three bears, with plenty left over.

melted coconut oil, for brushing

1½ cups rolled oats

½ cup chia seeds

½ cup shredded coconut

a pinch of salt

1 teaspoon ground ginger

½ teaspoon ground allspice

3 teaspoons ground cinnamon

2½ cups soy milk, plus extra to serve

4 tablespoons agave syrup,
  brown sugar or coconut sugar

2 teaspoons pure vanilla extract

1 ripe banana, mashed

½ cup chopped pitted dates

2 cups fresh or frozen berries,
  or chopped seasonal fruit

2 tablespoons raw sugar

- Preheat the oven to 200°C conventional, or 180°C fan-forced. Brush a 2 litre baking dish with melted coconut oil.

- In a large mixing bowl, combine the oats, chia seeds, shredded coconut, salt, ginger, allspice and 2 teaspoons of the cinnamon.

- In a separate bowl, combine the soy milk, agave syrup, vanilla, mashed banana, dates and 1½ cups of the berries. Add to the oat mixture and stir gently to combine.

- Pour into the prepared baking dish, then leave to sit for a few minutes to allow the chia seeds to soak up some of the milk. Scatter the remaining ½ cup of berries over the oats, pressing down gently to embed them. Mix the raw sugar and remaining cinnamon mixture together and sprinkle over the oat mixture.

- Pop into the oven and bake for 35–45 minutes, or until the oat mixture is golden on top. Remove from the oven and allow to cool for 5 minutes before serving.

- Serve with extra soy milk or yoghurt on the side, if desired.

Variations

- Use grated apple and extra mashed banana in place of the berries.

- Replace the agave syrup with marmalade for a burst of citrus flavour.

- Add some chopped walnuts or pecans for crunch and a protein punch.

- For a Turkish-inspired twist, add 1 teaspoon ground cardamom and a handful of chopped pistachios.

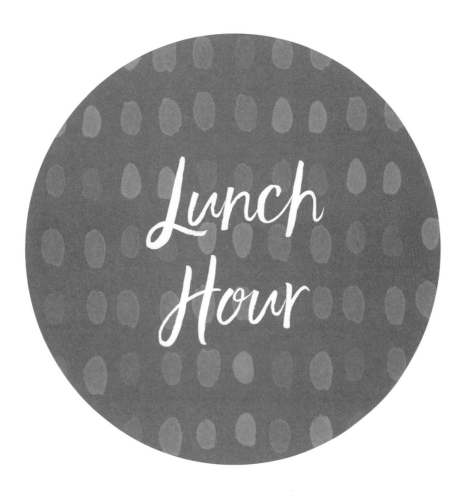

Lunch Hour

Throw together a sandwich on the run, share tacos with friends,
tuck into a hearty quiche for a summertime picnic or warm your
belly with a soul-satisfying soup in the depths of winter.
Make lunchtime interesting again – it's all here.

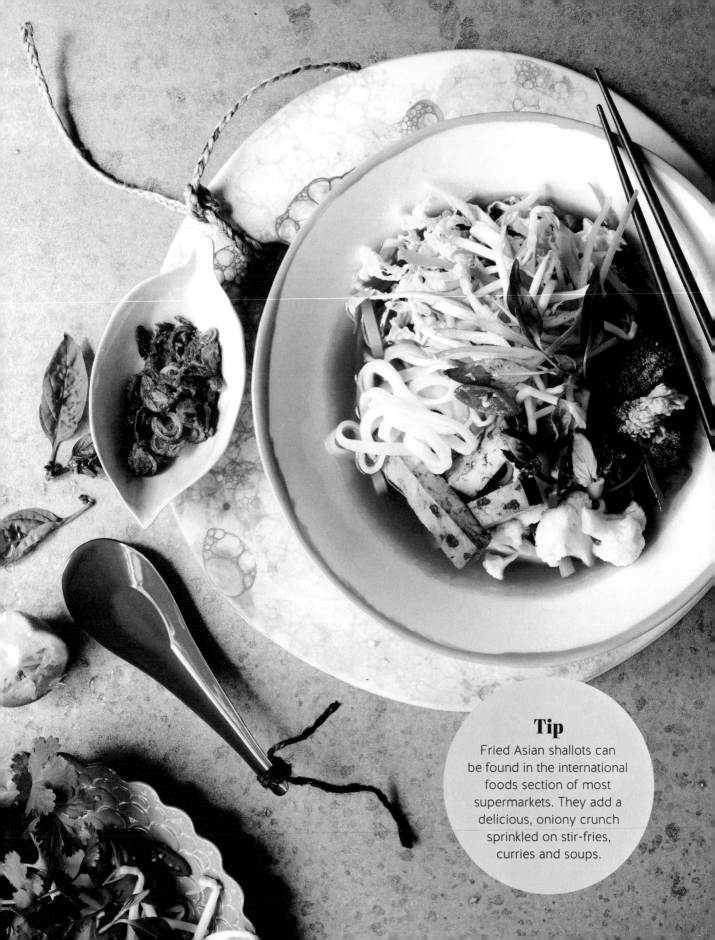

Tip

Fried Asian shallots can be found in the international foods section of most supermarkets. They add a delicious, oniony crunch sprinkled on stir-fries, curries and soups.

Ginger and Lemongrass Soup with Noodles

SERVES 4 GENEROUSLY

A build-your-own recipe, diners add herbs and seasonings to suit their own taste. This is a fun, hands-on dinner party recipe to share with loved ones and besties, because nothing says 'trust' like slurping up a bowl of slippery noodles in front of each other. The toppings are all optional, but a stack of serviettes is non-negotiable.

400–500 g dried flat rice noodles

1 teaspoon sesame oil

4 cups mixed vegetables, such as broccoli and cauliflower florets, peeled sliced carrots, trimmed green beans and shredded wombok cabbage

soy sauce, hoisin sauce and sriracha chilli sauce, to serve

LEMONGRASS BROTH

2 onions, unpeeled and quartered

5 cm piece fresh ginger, roughly chopped

2 cinnamon sticks

6 star anise (or less if you don't like a strong licorice flavour)

1 teaspoon whole coriander seeds

2 tablespoons rice bran oil

1 tablespoon sesame oil

4 garlic cloves, unpeeled and crushed

2 lemongrass stems, smashed, roughly chopped

2 teaspoons whole black peppercorns

2 celery stalks with leaves, roughly chopped

2 carrots, peeled, roughly chopped

1–3 tablespoons soy sauce or tamari

1–2 tablespoons hoisin sauce

2 teaspoons palm sugar

2 litres vegetable stock

8–12 fresh kaffir lime leaves, roughly torn

1 tablespoon lemon or lime juice

To make the broth, heat a large, heavy stockpot over medium–high heat. Add the onions and ginger to the dry pan and allow them to catch and caramelise slightly; this should take about 1 minute. Remove from the pan and set aside. In the same hot pan, dry fry the cinnamon sticks, star anise and coriander seeds for 30 seconds, or until roastily aromatic. Add the rice bran and sesame oils, then quickly stir in the onions and ginger again, along with the garlic cloves, lemongrass, peppercorns, celery and carrots. Stir constantly for 1 minute, before adding the soy sauce, hoisin sauce, palm sugar and stock. Add most of the kaffir lime leaves, setting some bits aside. Bring to the boil, then reduce the heat, cover and simmer for about 10–15 minutes.

Strain the soup through a fine colander, then return the liquid to the pan. Very finely shred the reserved kaffir lime leaf and add to the broth. Add the lemon or lime juice, then keep hot until ready to serve.

Prepare the noodles according to the packet instructions, then rinse with cold water, toss with the sesame oil, and set aside in a covered bowl until ready to serve.

Steam or microwave your chosen vegetables until just tender (wombok cabbage can be left raw). Blanch in cold water, then arrange on a platter. Arrange the garnish ingredients on the platter. Have the fried shallots, soy sauce, hoisin and sriracha and plenty of serviettes close at hand.

Bring the hot stockpot to the table and place on a wooden board. Divide the noodles evenly between four large, warmed bowls and allow people to add their chosen vegies before ladling in the piping-hot stock. Invite everyone to garnish and season their own bowls as desired.

TO GARNISH

1 batch Ginger and sesame tofu, cooked (page 111)

1 red onion, halved and finely sliced

4 spring onions, finely sliced

2 cups bean sprouts, rinsed

2 cups picked herbs, such as coriander, Vietnamese mint and Thai basil

fried Asian shallots (see tip), for sprinkling

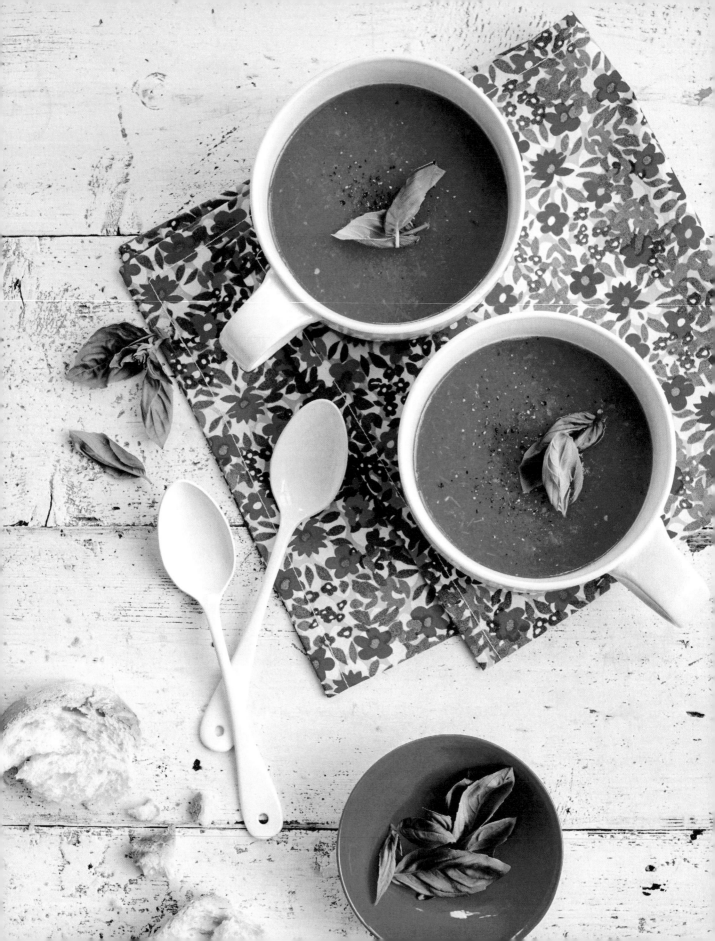

Roast Tomato and Capsicum Soup

SERVES 4-6

There's nothing quite like using whole roasted tomatoes for a hearty, homely soup to fill and warm your belly. This flavoursome soup is simple to prepare, and any leftovers can be refrigerated and are even tastier the next day. Serving the soup with fresh basil leaves helps bring out the rich flavours – and crusty bread is a must.

3 large red capsicums

1 kg tomatoes

2 large garlic cloves left unpeeled but crushed slightly

1 large brown onion, peeled and cut in half

1 large fennel bulb, cut in half

2 tablespoons olive oil

½ cup vegetable stock or water (optional)

a handful of basil leaves, torn

crusty bread, to serve

- Preheat the oven to 180°C conventional, or 160°C fan-forced. Line a large baking tray with baking paper.

- Cut the capsicums in half, then remove the membranes and seeds. Place the capsicums cut side down on the baking tray, along with the whole tomatoes, garlic cloves, and the onion and fennel halves. Drizzle with the olive oil, then roast in the oven for 1 hour, or until slightly browned. It's fine if the vegies catch and burn a little in patches – just call it 'caramelisation' and enjoy the added sweetness.

- When the vegetables are nicely roasted, transfer to a blender or food processor and blitz until smooth. There's no need to peel the tomatoes or capsicums – bonus!

- Pour the soup into a saucepan and slowly warm through over low heat. If the soup is too thick, slowly stir in the stock or water, until you reach the desired consistency. Season with salt and pepper to taste.

- Serve scattered with fresh basil, plenty of crusty bread on the side.

Tip

For a spicy 'Bloody Mary' flavour, add 3 finely diced celery stalks when frying the onion. Just before serving, add a few dashes of hot sauce and vegan Worcestershire sauce ... and if you want to add a shot of vodka as well, we won't tell!

Thai Pumpkin Soup

SERVES 4

*The subtle hints of green curry and coconut breathe new life into an old favourite.
This creamy, aromatic pumpkin soup is sure to be a go-to comfort food when autumn
rolls around. Serve with a big slice of toast, or over steamed basmati rice.*

1 tablespoon olive oil
1 brown onion, finely sliced
3 garlic cloves, sliced
2 tablespoons green curry
   paste (see tip)
½ butternut pumpkin (about
   700 g), peeled and chopped
   into 3 cm chunks
1 zucchini, grated
2 cups vegetable stock; add a little
   more if you prefer a thinner soup
270 ml coconut milk, approximately
a dash of soy sauce, to taste (optional)
chopped coriander, to serve

- Heat the olive oil in a large saucepan over medium heat and sauté the onion and garlic for about 5 minutes, until translucent. Stir in the green curry paste and cook for about 1 minute, taking care as it can splatter – there's nothing like an eyeful of chilli to ruin a perfectly good evening!

- Add the pumpkin and zucchini and stir well, ensuring the curry paste coats all the vegetables. Slowly pour in the stock and bring to the boil. Reduce the heat to a simmer and cook until the pumpkin is tender – this will take about 30–40 minutes.

- Remove from the heat and blend with a hand-held stick mixer until smooth – or wait until the soup has cooled and use a blender. If you like a thinner soup, add more water or stock at this point.

- Blend in half the coconut milk, adding more according to your taste. Season as required with salt, pepper, or a dash of soy sauce.

- Gently reheat the soup. Serve sprinkled with chopped coriander.

Tips

Be sure to look for
a fish-free, vegan green
curry paste! Butternut
pumpkin is especially lovely
in this soup on account
of its sweetness, but any
variety will work here.

Recipe contributed by Tiahn Wright

Spinach and Pumpkin Pasties

MAKES 8

*Filled with a creamy and comforting pumpkin filling, these golden pasties are great
with chutney. Mini versions make great appetisers, and also pack well for a picnic.
Larger pasties can be enjoyed as a simple supper with a crisp green salad.*

2 tablespoons olive oil, plus extra
  for brushing
1 teaspoon ground nutmeg
1 small or ½ large butternut pumpkin,
  peeled and cut into 1 cm cubes
2 small onions, thinly sliced
4 garlic cloves, peeled
250 g baby spinach leaves, chopped
250 g silken tofu
¼ cup soy sauce
2 sheets of frozen dairy-free puff
  pastry, thawed but still cold
soy milk, for brushing

Preheat the oven to 230°C conventional, or 210°C fan-forced. Line a large baking tray with baking paper.

In a bowl, mix together the olive oil and nutmeg. Add the pumpkin and onion and toss to coat, then place on the baking tray, along with the whole garlic cloves. Roast for 20–25 minutes, or until a knife slides easily into the pumpkin. Remove from the oven and set aside to cool for about 20 minutes.

Put the spinach and tofu in a large bowl and mix together, squishing the tofu up a bit. Drizzle with the soy sauce and season with salt and pepper. Mash the cooled pumpkin, onion and garlic together, then fold through the spinach mixture.

Cut the pastry sheets into quarters. Spoon about 2 tablespoons of the pumpkin filling into one corner of each pastry square, taking care not to add too much filling, or the pasties may burst open in the oven. Fold each quarter diagonally over the filling, to form a triangle. Dab the edges with olive oil, then press together to seal. Now make a few little snips with kitchen scissors or the tip of a knife to create steam holes, so the pasties don't burst open during baking.

Place your pasties on one or two baking trays lined with baking paper, then brush the tops with a little soy milk for extra golden-brown goodness. Bake for 20–30 minutes, until the pastry is golden and puffy.

Serve warm.

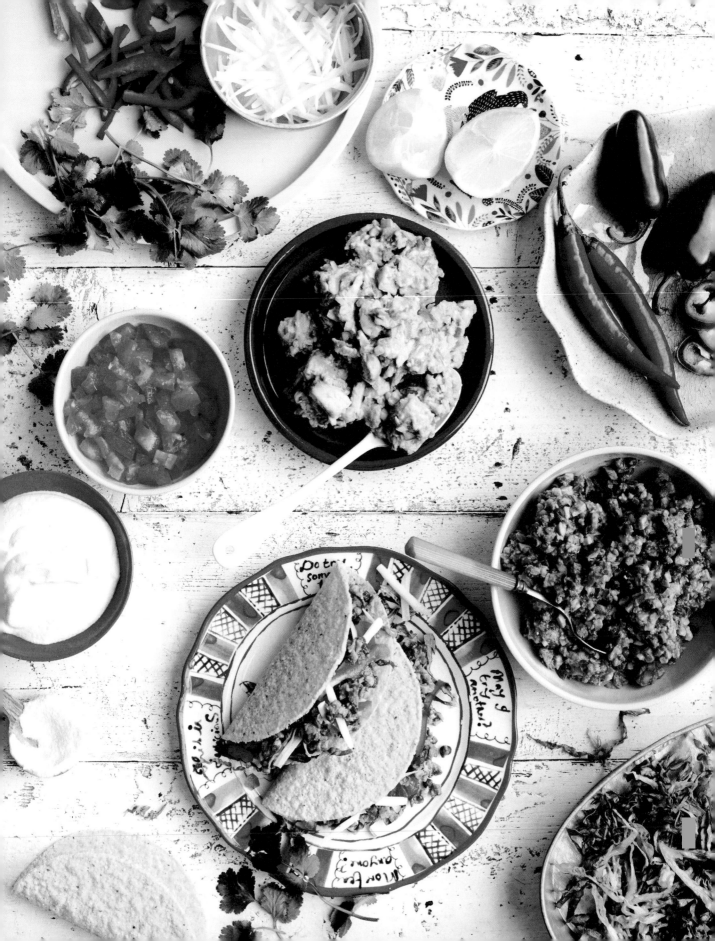

Spicy Lentil and Walnut Tacos

SERVES 4

This healthy variation on the traditional mince taco boasts an incredible texture thanks to the surprising binding quality of ground walnuts. Great as a fresh summer treat and packed full of vegie goodness, it's a surprisingly low-fuss and high-protein win! For a lighter lunch option, use cos lettuce leaves instead of taco shells.

500 g button mushrooms

½ cup walnuts

2 tablespoons olive oil

½ onion, finely diced

1 garlic clove, crushed

1 teaspoon chilli flakes

1–2 x 28 g sachets taco seasoning, or homemade seasoning (see tip)

400 g tin lentils, rinsed and drained

8 taco shells

TACO TOPPINGS

1 cup Guacamole (page 163)

1 cup Cashew sour cream (page 159)

3 cups finely shredded iceberg lettuce

2 cups diced tomatoes

1 cup finely sliced red capsicum

1 cup grated dairy-free cheese

½ cup chopped coriander, for garnishing

- Finely chop the mushrooms into tiny cubes, and use a food processor to grind the walnuts into a coarse powder. Set aside.

- In a saucepan, heat the olive oil over medium heat. Fry the onion, garlic and chilli flakes for 5 minutes, until the onion is translucent and aromatic. Add the chopped mushrooms and fry for a further 5 minutes, stirring occasionally, until they begin to soften. Stir in the taco seasoning and ½ cup water and simmer for 30 seconds.

- Stir the lentils into the mushroom mixture, along with the ground walnuts. Cook, stirring, for 2 minutes, or until the mixture thickens. Remove from the heat and keep warm until ready to serve.

- Meanwhile, heat the taco shells according to the packet instructions.

- Place all the taco toppings in separate bowls, including the hot lentil and walnut filling, and the hot taco shells. Serve straight away, inviting diners to fill their own tacos however they choose.

Tip

To make your own taco seasoning, combine 1 teaspoon each onion and garlic powder, 1 teaspoon chilli flakes, 2 teaspoons dried oregano, 1 tablespoon hot or sweet paprika, 2 teaspoons ground cumin and some salt and pepper.

Cauliflower Buffalo 'Wings'

MAKES 4 SMALL SERVINGS

These South Western–style buffalo 'wings' make an awesomely tasty fuss-free lunch when you're expecting friends around; they're also great as a starter, snack or side dish. The cauliflower offers a meaty texture, complemented by a crispy, spicy coating of batter and a creamy ranch-style dipping sauce. The 'wings' take a little while to bake, but are otherwise super quick and simple to toss together.

¾ cup plain flour; for a gluten-free option, try rice flour or chickpea flour (besan)

¼ teaspoon sea salt

¼ teaspoon black pepper

1½ teaspoons garlic powder

2 teaspoons onion powder

1 teaspoon ground cumin

1 teaspoon smoked, hot or sweet paprika

½ cup unsweetened dairy-free milk, such as almond or soy milk

1 head of cauliflower, cut into bite-sized florets

1 tablespoon dairy-free margarine

2 tablespoons hot sauce, such as chilli or sriracha

1 cup barbecue sauce

Creamy ranch dressing (page 161), to serve

- Preheat the oven to 250°C conventional, or 230°C fan-forced. Line two baking trays with baking paper.

- In a bowl, combine the flour, salt, pepper and other ground spices. Pour in the milk and ½ cup water and whisk until smooth. The consistency of the batter is important: it shouldn't be so thick that it doesn't drip, but also not so thin that it won't coat or stick to the cauliflower. If you're using rice or chickpea flour, you may need a little more liquid for optimal consistency.

- Dip each cauliflower floret into the batter, coating them evenly. Tap off the excess batter a few times on the side of the bowl, then place the florets on the lined baking trays, laying them out evenly.

- Bake for 15 minutes, then flip the florets over and bake for another 10 minutes, or until golden brown and crispy.

- While the cauliflower is baking, place the margarine, hot sauce and barbecue sauce in a saucepan over low heat. Remove from the heat just as the margarine starts melting. Stir together and set aside.

- Remove the crispy cauliflower from the oven and place in a large mixing bowl with the hot barbecue sauce mix. Toss to coat evenly. (If your bowl isn't quite large enough, this may need to be done in several batches.)

- Spread the florets out on the same baking trays and bake for a further 20–25 minutes, flipping the florets over halfway through.

- When the desired crispiness is achieved, remove the florets from the oven. Serve warm, with the Creamy ranch dressing as a dipping sauce.

Recipe contributed by hot for food

Vietnamese Rice Paper Rolls

SERVES 4 AS A STARTER

A fresh, fragrant twist on deep-fried spring rolls, these Vietnamese rice paper rolls are packed with aromatic herbs, crunchy vegies and protein-rich tofu, and are perfect for picnics and lunchboxes.

75–100 g dried rice vermicelli noodles

1 Lebanese cucumber

1 carrot, peeled

1 small red capsicum

2 spring onions

1 avocado

a squeeze of lemon juice

2 cups mixed fresh herbs, such as basil, mint, coriander and Vietnamese mint

8 large round rice paper sheets

1 serve of Ginger and sesame tofu (page 111), pan-fried

1 serve of Satay sauce (from the Vegetable kebabs on page 139)

- Prepare the noodles according to the packet instructions; you should end up with 1–1½ cups cooked noodles. Set aside while you prepare all the gorgeous fresh vegies.

- Basically, you're aiming to get all your vegies to the same size. Thinly slice the cucumber, carrot, capsicum and spring onions lengthways. Slice the avocado flesh into long strips, then quickly sprinkle with lemon juice to stop it browning. Pick the leaves off the herbs, rinse well to get rid of any grit, then pat dry with a clean tea towel.

- Fill a bowl with some warm water, then slide a single sheet of rice paper into the water. Leave for just a minute or so, until it turns pliable and somewhat translucent, then carefully remove and place on a clean and slightly damp tea towel.

- Place about a tablespoon of the noodles into the middle of the softened rice paper sheet. Layer with a small portion of the tofu, vegies and herbs. Fold in the sides of the rice paper, like you're making a burrito or tucking someone into bed, then firmly roll up, tucking the ends in as you go. (If you need a visual guide, there are heaps of videos on the internet!)

- Repeat with the remaining rice paper sheets and fillings. Pack the Vietnamese rice paper rolls into an airtight container and keep refrigerated until ready to eat.

- Serve with the satay sauce for dipping.

Tip

Instead of satay sauce, you can serve these rolls with a small bowl of vegan hoisin dipping sauce, which has been sprinkled with some crushed peanuts and finely chopped red chilli.

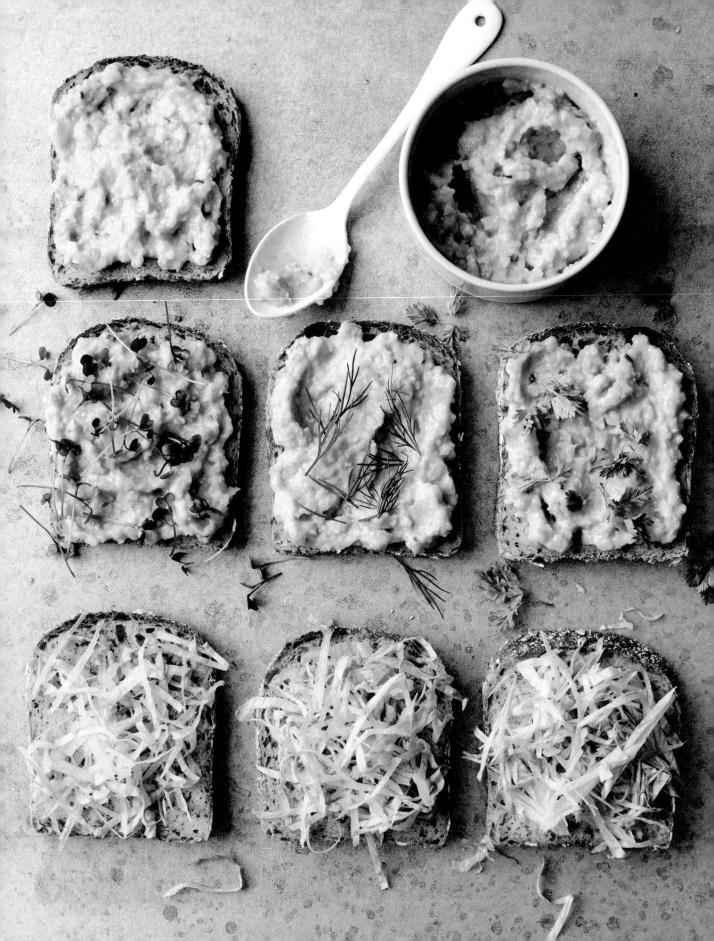

Tangy Chicky Tuna-less Sandwiches

MAKES 4-6

*With a light and versatile filling, these sandwiches are perfect for daily lunches
or picnics, or cut into fingers for a dainty high tea. The addition of nori sushi sheets,
while optional, gives the filling a delightfully briny, salty flavour.*

8-12 slices of fresh wholegrain bread
shredded iceberg lettuce, to serve
fresh herbs (optional), to serve

CHICKY TUNA-LESS FILLING

400 g tin chickpeas, rinsed
    and drained
¼ cup egg-free mayonnaise
½ teaspoon dijon or wholegrain
    mustard
2 tablespoons lemon juice
1 tablespoon olive oil
½ cup chopped celery
2 chives, finely chopped
2 teaspoons baby capers, drained
a pinch of cayenne pepper
¼ cup chopped dill
1 teaspoon chia seeds (optional)
1 tablespoon tamari or soy sauce
2 toasted nori sheets, shredded
    (optional)

Place all the filling ingredients in a blender or food processor. Season with salt and pepper to taste. Pulse for no longer than 30 seconds in total, checking intermittently that the mixture isn't turning into a paste. You're aiming for a rough mash, so it's fine if some chickpeas remain almost whole. (You could also do this the old-fashioned way and squash all the ingredients together with a potato masher.)

Spread the mixture over half the bread slices. Top with shredded lettuce, and some fresh herbs if using, sandwich the other bread slices on top and serve straight away.

Variations

- Make a melt by layering the filling with a few slices of dairy-free cheese. Pop the sandwich in a toasted-sandwich maker, or fry in a frying pan with a little splash of oil over medium heat until golden brown.

- Add some mashed avocado, grated carrot or a sprinkling of pine nuts or sunflower seeds to the mixture, for extra flavour and nutrition.

Curried Egg-less Sandwiches

MAKES 8 SANDWICHES

You'll never look at tofu the same way again – and neither will your guests! Here it transforms into a soft and lightly curried filling that is healthy, delicious and 100% chicken-friendly. These sandwiches travel well, so next time you're going on a picnic or road trip, whip up a batch of these. We recommend doubling the recipe if you're picnicking – what is it about eating outdoors that makes people ravenous?

16 slices of white bread

CURRIED EGG-LESS FILLING

250 g firm tofu, drained, squeezed
   dry and crumbled
1 medium potato, cooked, mashed
   and cooled
½ onion, finely chopped
¼ cup egg-free mayonnaise
2 tablespoons curry powder
2 teaspoons ground turmeric
1½ celery stalks, finely chopped
3 garlic cloves, crushed
2–3 tablespoons chopped parsley
   or chives (optional)

- In a large bowl, mix all the filling ingredients together. Season with salt to taste.
- Spread the filling onto half the bread slices. Sandwich the other bread slices on top, cut in half and serve!
- If you're taking the sandwiches to a picnic or on a road trip, keep the filling and the bread separate and make the sandwiches just before serving, so the bread doesn't go soggy.

Tips

For a creamier texture, add a little more mayonnaise. Instead of celery, try finely chopped spinach, chard or silverbeet – or layer with some shredded cos lettuce for added crunch.

Tomato and Spinach Quiche

SERVES 6-8

Quiche as you've never known it before – soft and fluffy, packed with layers of juicy cherry tomatoes, fried mushrooms and sweet caramelised onion. But don't feel bound by the vegetables used here: experiment with other wonderful additions, such as olives, sundried tomatoes, asparagus and artichokes.

1 red capsicum
8 large cherry tomatoes, cut in half
1 tablespoon olive oil
1 red onion, sliced
2 teaspoons balsamic vinegar
1 tablespoon brown sugar
10 button mushrooms, sliced
1½ sheets of frozen dairy-free shortcrust pastry, thawed
1 loosely packed cup baby spinach leaves

GLORIOUSLY GOLDEN QUICHE FILLING

¼ cup self-raising flour
½ cup chickpea flour (besan)
2 tablespoons nutritional yeast
½ teaspoon Indian black salt (from Indian grocery stores; also called kala namak or sanchal), or sea salt
1 teaspoon onion powder
1 teaspoon garlic powder
2 teaspoons ground turmeric
600 g firm silken tofu
100 g dairy-free cheese, grated

- Preheat the oven to 230°C conventional, or 210°C fan-forced.
- To make the filling, place the self-raising flour, chickpea flour, nutritional yeast, salt and ground spices in a food processor. Briefly blend together, then add the tofu and cheese and process until smooth. Set aside.
- To roast the capsicum, bake for 30 minutes. Leave to sweat in a plastic bag for 10 minutes, then peel away the skin. The cherry tomatoes can also be roasted at the same time, for about 15 minutes.
- Heat the olive oil in a frying pan. Add the onion and sauté over medium-high heat for about 5 minutes, stirring occasionally, until it begins to brown. Turn the heat down low and cook for a further 15 minutes, stirring now and then. Stir in the balsamic vinegar and sugar and cook for a further 10–15 minutes, until the onion is sweet and glossy. Scrape into a bowl and set aside.
- Add the mushrooms to the same frying pan (they'll soak up any residual sweetness from the caramelised onion). Turn the heat up to medium-high and cook, stirring occasionally, for about 5 minutes, or until lightly browned. Set aside to cool.
- Press the pastry into the base and side of a greased 25 cm flan tin. Cover with baking paper and place baking beads or dry rice or beans on top. Bake for 10 minutes. (This stage is known as blind-baking, and will ensure your quiche doesn't have a soggy pastry base.)
- Spread the caramelised onion over the pastry base, then cover with a thin layer of the filling mixture. Add the mushrooms, tomatoes, capsicum and spinach leaves, spacing them evenly so each slice of quiche will have a bit of everything.
- Cover with the remaining filling, then pop in the oven for about 30 minutes, until lightly browned on top. Remove from the oven and allow to stand for a few minutes, before slicing and serving to your adoring fans.
- This quiche is also fabulous cold, and makes excellent picnic fodder.

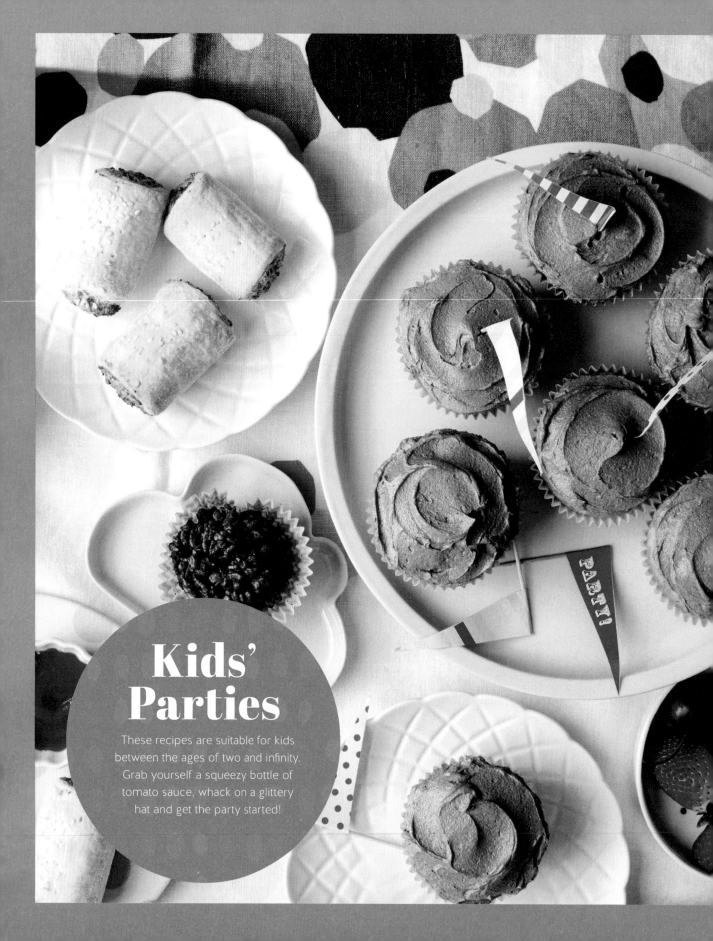

Kids' Parties

These recipes are suitable for kids
between the ages of two and infinity.
Grab yourself a squeezy bottle of
tomato sauce, whack on a glittery
hat and get the party started!

Vanilla Cupcakes with Fluffy Chocolate Icing

MAKES 12-14 CUPCAKES

Dainty bites of deliciousness, with that perfect indentation when you peel away the paper patty case. These will be a hit at kids' parties (especially with some sprinkles on top!), school fund-raisers, or as an after-dinner treat.

2 cups plain flour
1 cup sugar
2 teaspoons baking powder
1 teaspoon bicarbonate of soda
½ teaspoon salt
1 teaspoon finely grated lemon zest
   (optional)
1½ cups dairy-free milk
½ cup coconut yoghurt
1 tablespoon dairy-free margarine
1 tablespoon apple cider vinegar
2 teaspoons pure vanilla extract
½ cup sunflower or coconut oil

FLUFFY CHOCOLATE ICING

1 cup dairy-free margarine
2 teaspoons pure vanilla extract
2 tablespoons cocoa powder
3 cups icing sugar mixture,
   approximately

- Preheat the oven to 180°C conventional, or 160°C fan-forced. Line a cupcake tray or muffin tray with paper cases.
- In a bowl, combine the flour, sugar, baking powder, bicarbonate of soda, salt and lemon zest, if using. Mix well, then add the remaining cake ingredients. Using a high-speed blender, mix together until the mixture is smooth and free of any lumps.
- Spoon the batter into the paper cases, filling them roughly two-thirds full.
- Bake for 20 minutes, or until the cakes spring back when gently pressed. Remove from the oven and leave to cool before icing.
- To make the icing, place the margarine and vanilla in a bowl, add a tiny pinch of salt and beat together using an electric mixer until whipped and nicely creamy. Sieve the cocoa powder and half the icing sugar mixture over the top and mix well. Start your beaters on slow, then gradually speed up, so you don't end up with powder all over your kitchen.
- Gradually sieve another cup of the icing sugar mixture over the top, beating it in well. Taste test time! If you like your icing sweeter, add the rest of the icing sugar and beat again until well combined.
- Pipe or spoon the icing onto your cooled cupcakes and enjoy.
- These cupcakes are best served the same day they are made, but will keep in the fridge in an airtight container for several days.

Variation: For a 'jaffa'-style icing, add the finely grated zest of 1 orange when beating the margarine and vanilla together.

'Sausage' Rolls

MAKES 40 MINI ROLLS

These bite-sized crunchy, golden rolls of filled pastry are a perennial favourite of kids and grown-ups alike.

5 sheets of frozen dairy-free
   puff pastry
100 g pecans
4 slices of bread (about 100 g)
1 brown onion, roughly chopped
1 teaspoon garlic powder
1 teaspoon onion powder
¼ teaspoon freshly ground
   black pepper
1 teaspoon vegan beef-style
   stock powder
1 teaspoon dried thyme
1 small bunch flat-leaf parsley
1 tablespoon soy sauce
250 g silken tofu
tomato sauce, to serve (optional)

- Preheat the oven to 230°C conventional, or 210°C fan-forced. Line two baking trays with baking paper.
- Remove the pastry sheets from the freezer to thaw.
- Briefly blend the pecans in a food processor, leaving them a little coarse for a bit of texture; be careful not to overprocess or they will turn into a paste. Set aside in a bowl.
- Process the bread until it turns into crumbs, then add to the nut mixture.
- Blend the onion, spices, stock powder, herbs, soy sauce and tofu until combined, then add to the nut mixture and mix well.
- The pastry sheets should be thawed by now; if not, separate the sheets and place on a flat surface and they will thaw very quickly. Cut each pastry sheet in half to make two long pieces. Put a line of the nut mixture, 2–3 cm thick, 2 cm in from the pastry edge. Fold the pastry over the mixture and press down. Use a fork to seal along the edge, then roll up into a tube. Cut each long roll into four mini rolls.
- Place the rolls on the baking trays and bake for 30 minutes, or until the pastry is golden brown. Serve warm, with tomato sauce if desired.

Fairy Bread

SERVES 10

What kids' party would be complete without these yummy rainbow-coloured treats? Keep them simple, or join in the fun by using cookie cutters to cut the fairy bread into special shapes the kids will love. You could even decorate some of them with dairy-free chocolate sprinkles!

1 loaf of soft white bread
dairy-free margarine, for spreading
hundreds and thousands,
   for sprinkling

- Remove the crusts from the bread, if desired. Spread the bread slices with margarine.
- Shake the hundreds and thousands over the slices, then cut each slice into triangles, smaller squares or other shapes that take your fancy.
- Arrange on plates and serve straight away.

Pita Scrolls

Don't be fooled by the sneaky greens: kids love these pita scrolls. If preparing them a few hours before serving, use a light hand with the hummus and sweet chilli sauce, so the scrolls don't become soggy.

8 thin 'mountain bread'-style pita breads

200 g tub of hummus (or use your favourite home-made version)

2 cups grated carrot, squeezed in paper towels to remove excess moisture

2 avocados, halved, pitted and thinly sliced

1 cup baby spinach leaves, washed and dried

sweet chilli sauce, for drizzling

- Arrange 4 of the pita bread sheets on a clean work surface. Stack another pita bread sheet on top of each, to make four double stacks. (Using a double layer of pita gives the scrolls more structure and minimises sogginess.) Spread the top sheets with a thin layer of hummus, leaving a 1 cm gap along one side, so it doesn't squish out the edges when you roll it up. Leaving the same gap, and keeping the layers of fillings thin to allow for firm rolling, arrange the grated carrot, avocado slices and baby spinach over the pitas. Drizzle each lightly with sweet chilli sauce.

- One at a time, gently but firmly roll up each pita stack and place on a clean chopping board, with the pita join facing the bottom. Use a sharp knife to cut each roll into 5 slices, creating bite-sized scrolls.

- Use toothpicks to secure each scroll, before carefully transferring to a serving platter or plates, using a spatula if needed. Remember to remove the toothpicks before serving. Serve immediately, or cover and chill in the fridge for no more than 3 hours.

Variations: Instead of hummus, use dairy-free cream cheese, nut butter or other vegan dips (pages 154–163); thinly sliced pitted olives, sundried tomatoes, sultanas or pineapple pieces can add interest. Instead of sweet chilli sauce, drizzle with tomato or barbecue sauce.

Chocolate Crackles

Crispy and chocolatey, this old-school favourite is popular for a reason. What more could you want from a party food? For extra fun, add 3 tablespoons of hundreds and thousands before stirring the melted chocolate through.

3½ cups puffed rice cereal

½ cup shredded or desiccated coconut

100 g dairy-free dark chocolate

100 g dairy-free milk chocolate

- Combine the puffed rice and coconut in a large mixing bowl and mix until combined. Set out 12 paper cases on a tray.

- Melt the dark and milk chocolate together in a small saucepan over medium-low heat, stirring regularly. When melted, pour over the dry ingredients and mix together well. Spoon the mixture into the paper cases. Chill in the fridge for 1 hour, or until set.

- This mixture also works well if pressed firmly into a rectangular baking tin, refrigerated, then sliced into bars or squares.

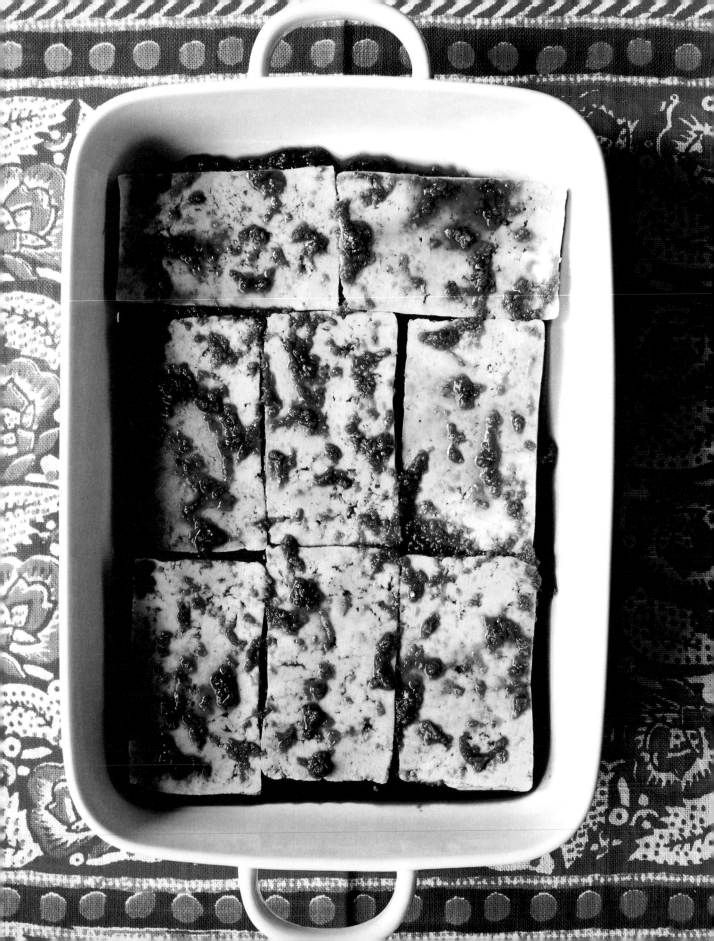

Ginger and Sesame Tofu

SERVES 2

Here's a simple, flavoursome, versatile way with tofu. You can bake or pan-fry the marinated tofu and use it as a sandwich filling with salad, toss the marinated tofu through a stir-fry, or skewer it with some onion and red capsicum chunks and grill it on the barbecue. It's worth marinating a larger batch, as it will keep in the fridge for a few days to use as a base for a multitude of quick and tasty meals.

375 g packet firm tofu (a little more or less is fine)

¼ cup soy sauce or tamari

3 garlic cloves, crushed

2 cm piece fresh ginger, peeled and grated

a few drops of sesame oil

- Slice the tofu thinly, then pack into a sandwich bag or fridge-safe container.

- Mix together the soy sauce, garlic, ginger and sesame oil, then pour over the tofu. Toss the tofu slices to ensure they're well coated in the sauce mixture, then marinate in the fridge for at least 1 hour, or up to a few days.

- The tofu can be cooked in so many ways: stir-fried, pan-fried, barbecued, or baked at 180°C for 15 minutes. Serve hot.

Tips

The soy ginger marinade is also delicious with tempeh.

Try serving with a sprinkling of sesame seeds, chilli flakes or chopped spring onions.

Spicy Potato Wedges

SERVES 4

What is it about hot, crunchy, crispy potatoes that makes us want to devour the lot? Do we have some kind of special second stomach (closely related to the well-known 'dessert stomach') that is purely there to fill with potato goodness? The answer may be beyond our grasp – but thankfully, these spicy wedges are not! We love these with egg-free mayo and sweet chilli sauce.

3 teaspoons salt

1 kg waxy potatoes, such as nicola, kipfler or golden delight, unpeeled but washed well and cut into wedges

100 ml olive oil

½ teaspoon freshly ground black pepper

1–2 tablespoons sweet paprika

½ teaspoon cayenne pepper or chilli flakes (optional)

1 teaspoon garlic powder

1 teaspoon onion powder

½ teaspoon dried oregano

½ teaspoon dried thyme

½ teaspoon dried sage

½ teaspoon dried basil (see tip)

Preheat the oven to 210°C conventional, or 190°C fan-forced. Pop a roasting tin inside to warm.

Bring a large pot of water to the boil. Add 2 teaspoons of the salt, stir, then carefully drop in the potato wedges. Boil for about 10 minutes, or until the potatoes are just tender all the way through when pierced with a skewer.

Drain the potatoes in a colander. Give them a bit of a shake to rough up the outside into a fluffy coating – but not so hard that you end up with a sink full of mashed potato. Set aside to air dry for a few minutes while you prepare the rest of the ingredients.

Put the remaining 1 teaspoon salt in a small bowl. Add ⅓ cup of the olive oil, along with all the spices and dried herbs, and mix together well.

Wearing oven mitts, remove the roasting tin from the oven and drizzle in the remaining olive oil. Swirl around to coat the base, then add the potatoes. They might sizzle a bit, so lean back when you tip them in!

Drizzle the potatoes with the spiced oil mixture and stir gently to coat. Slide the pan back into the oven and roast for about 15 minutes.

Remove the pan from the oven and, using a spatula, flip the potatoes over to roast the other side. Bake for another 5–10 minutes, until crispy. Serve immediately.

Tips

Don't omit the dried basil. For some reason it adds magic here.

For Mexican-style wedges, add 1 teaspoon ground cumin to the spice mixture and top the hot wedges with chopped fresh coriander. Olé!

Cauliflower Soup with Garlic Bread

SERVES 8

Soup is a delicious way to enjoy cauliflower. This recipe is not only super easy, but super creamy too. Cumin imparts a subtle nuttiness that pairs fabulously well with garlic bread – but if you really want to shake things up, add a tablespoon or two of your favourite curry powder as well. Cauliflower and curry go together like Doctor Who and the TARDIS, transcending time and space.

3 tablespoons olive oil
2 large red onions, chopped
3 garlic cloves, chopped
1 tablespoon ground cumin
3 large potatoes, chopped
   (peeled or unpeeled)
1 cauliflower, roughly chopped
1 bay leaf
4 cups vegetable stock

GARLIC BREAD
2–3 tablespoons dairy-free margarine
1–3 garlic cloves, crushed
pinch of dried Italian herb mix
¾ teaspoon salt
1 baguette

Heat the olive oil in a large saucepan over medium heat. Add the onion and sauté for about 5 minutes, until translucent. Add the garlic and cumin and sauté for a further 2 minutes.

Now add the potato, cauliflower, bay leaf and stock. Pour in 3 cups water, or enough water so that the liquid almost covers the vegetables. Bring to the boil, then reduce the heat and simmer for about 20 minutes, or until the vegetables are soft. Set aside to cool slightly.

Remove the bay leaf, then use a stick blender to process until smooth. Season with salt and pepper to taste, gently reheat and serve.

Preheat the oven to 220°C conventional, or 200°C fan-forced.

To make the garlic bread, mix together the margarine, garlic, dried Italian herb mix and salt. Cut the baguette into 2 cm slices. Evenly spread the garlic margarine over each slice, put the baguette back together and wrap the whole thing in foil. Pop into the oven for 10–12 minutes, then it's ready to devour.

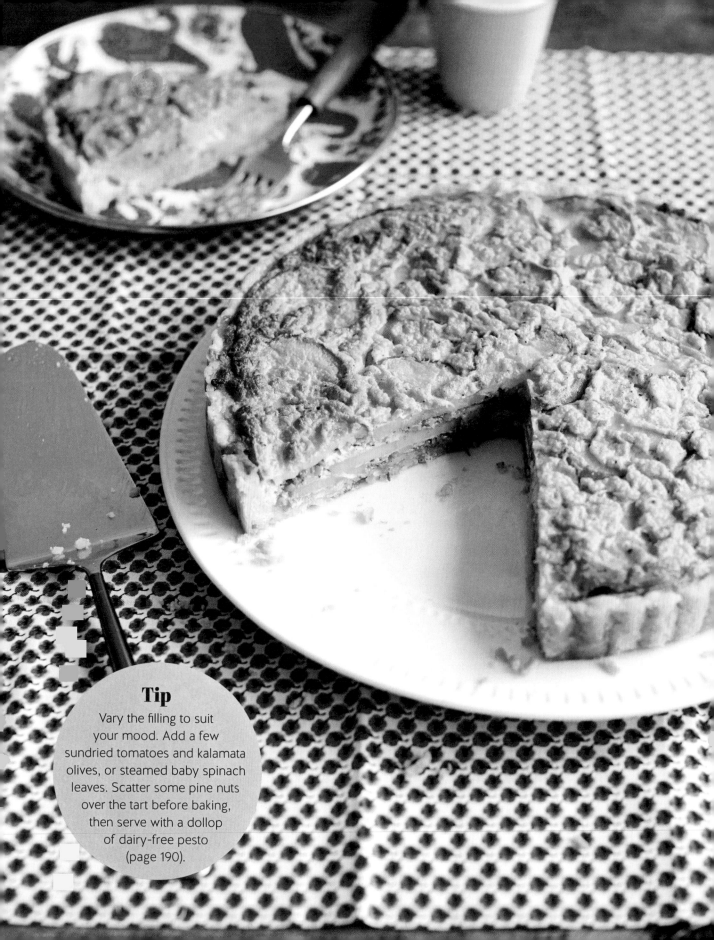

Tip

Vary the filling to suit your mood. Add a few sundried tomatoes and kalamata olives, or steamed baby spinach leaves. Scatter some pine nuts over the tart before baking, then serve with a dollop of dairy-free pesto (page 190).

Potato and Leek Tart

SERVES 4 GENEROUSLY

*We think this will be the start of a delicious relationship, where leek and potato soup
meets pie – resulting in a culinary romance in which a creamy, intensely flavoured filling is enclosed
by a simple, foolproof pastry shell. Perfect for every occasion, from picnics to dinner parties.*

⅔ cup plain flour
½ cup self-raising flour
½ cup cornflour
½–1 teaspoon salt
½–⅔ cup coconut oil, set solid
    (if yours is liquid, just chill it
    in the fridge for 15 minutes)
1 tablespoon dairy-free milk, chilled

POTATO AND LEEK FILLING

3 medium potatoes, sliced no thicker
    than 3 mm (to make 2 cups)
1 tablespoon olive oil
2 leeks, pale section only, sliced no
    thicker than 3 mm (to make 2 cups)
½ teaspoon salt
½ teaspoon dried oregano or dried
    thyme (or both!)
1 teaspoon dried sage
3 garlic cloves, crushed
2 teaspoons vegan beef-style
    stock powder
2 tablespoons dairy-free milk
500 g silken tofu
½ teaspoon ground turmeric
1 teaspoon garlic powder
1 teaspoon onion powder
½ teaspoon freshly ground
    black pepper
2 tablespoons nutritional yeast
1 tablespoon self-raising flour
1 tablespoon cornflour

- Preheat the oven to 200°C conventional, or 180°C fan-forced. Dig out a 24 cm tart tin with a fluted edge – a non-stick one with a removable base is ideal. (You can also use a spring-form cake tin, but your tart edges may not end up as neat.)

- Now, let's make some pastry. Sift the plain flour, self-raising flour, cornflour and salt together into a bowl, then rub in the solid coconut oil with the tips of your fingers. You're aiming for a texture that looks roughly like breadcrumbs, but some bigger lumps are perfectly fine. (If the coconut oil is very hard, you can grate it in to start with, dipping the coconut oil in flour to avoid gunking up your grater.)

- Add just enough cold milk, a teaspoon at a time, to hold the mixture together – it doesn't matter if it's a bit crumbly. Press the pastry into your tart tin, and all the way up the side, as evenly as you can. Pop it in the fridge while you get on with the filling.

- Firstly, steam or microwave your potato slices until they're just cooked, then set aside. Meanwhile, warm the olive oil in a frying pan over medium heat, then add the leek and salt. Cook, stirring occasionally, for 7–10 minutes, or until the leek has softened. Add the oregano, sage, garlic and 1 teaspoon of the stock powder and stir to combine. Cook for a further 30 seconds, then stir in 1 tablespoon of the milk and deglaze the pan. Remove from the heat and set aside.

- Now pop your pastry-lined tin in the oven and precook it for 10 minutes.

- Meanwhile, place the tofu, turmeric, garlic powder, onion powder, pepper, nutritional yeast, flour and cornflour in a blender. Add the remaining 1 tablespoon of milk and 1 teaspoon of stock powder and blitz for about 20 seconds, or until the ingredients are combined.

- Remove the pastry from the oven. Begin layering the filling, starting with a few spoonfuls of the leek, then a layer of potato slices, then a layer of the tofu mixture. Keep going until you run out of ingredients, or reach the top of the tin, making sure you finish with a layer of the tofu mixture.

- Return to the oven and bake for 30 minutes, or until the top feels set when pressed lightly with your fingers; the filling will continue to cook a little as the tart cools.

- Remove from the oven. If serving warm, leave to cool a little before carefully removing from the tin.

Vegie Soup

SERVES 4, WITH LEFTOVERS FOR LUNCH THE NEXT DAY

Its simple name disguises just how comforting this colourful and nourishing soup is. Wholesome and reliable, it features a surprise ingredient that does a delicious job of binding this whole 'hug in a mug' meal together: creamed corn. Don't knock it 'til you try it!

2 tablespoons olive oil

2 large golden onions, diced

1 leek, pale section only, halved and cut into thin half-moons

4 celery stalks, thinly sliced

4 large carrots, peeled and grated

1–2 tablespoons mild curry powder

3–4 large waxy or boiling potatoes, peeled and cut into large dice

½ large kent pumpkin, peeled and cut into large dice

2 zucchini, cut into bite-sized pieces (optional)

1 tablespoon vegan beef-style stock powder

1 teaspoon ground turmeric

2 teaspoons whole black peppercorns

400 g tin creamed corn

a large handful of roughly chopped parsley

Warm a large heavy-based saucepan over medium heat. Add the olive oil, onions, leek, celery, carrots, curry powder and a pinch of salt. Cover and cook, stirring occasionally, for a few minutes, until the onion is translucent.

Add the potatoes, pumpkin and zucchini, if using. Stir in a splash of water if the vegies are starting to stick. Cover the pan to create a little sauna, then leave the vegetables to sweat for about 5 minutes.

Give everything a stir, then add the stock powder, turmeric and peppercorns. Pour in a little water – just enough to reach below the top of the vegetables. (They will continue releasing juices as they cook, and you don't want the soup to be too thin; you can always add more water later.)

Bring the soup up to a boil, then reduce the heat to a slow simmer. Cover and cook for 1¼ hours, or until the potatoes are tender, stirring occasionally to ensure the vegies cook evenly.

Stir in the creamed corn and simmer for a further 15 minutes.

Just before serving, stir through the parsley, so it retains its lovely fresh colour and aroma.

Tip

For an even heartier meal, add your favourite tinned beans when adding the creamed corn. Kidney beans, chickpeas and butterbeans work particularly well. Rinse and drain them before adding to the soup.

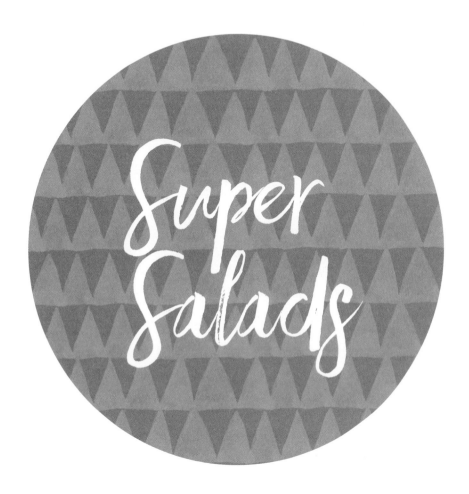

Super Salads

Gone are the days of limp iceberg with a tomato slice. It's time to rethink and reinvent salads – with noodles, potatoes, black rice, roasted vegies and more. Don't banish your salad to a sad side dish – let these gourmet super salads shine as the main star of your meal.

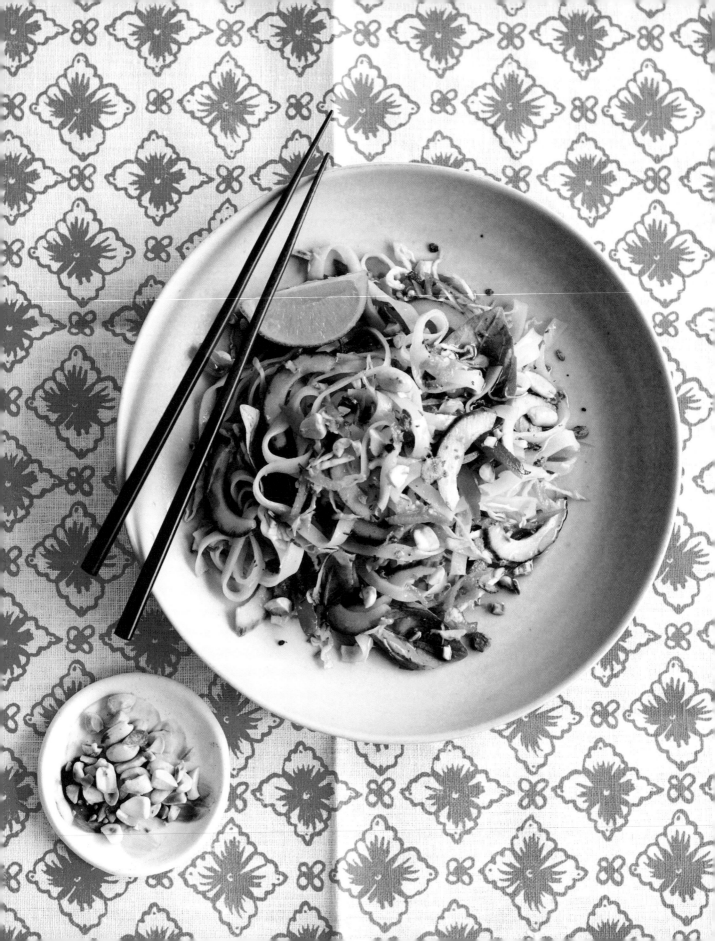

Fragrant Cambodian Noodle Salad

MAKES 2 LARGE OR 4 SMALL SERVES

Light, fragrant and sweet … this has everything you want in a noodle salad. It's quick to make, and is packed full of goodness for a filling feed and long-lasting fuel for your body. For a more substantial meal, serve with Sticky BBQ tofu (page 141). Top with thinly sliced red chilli if you like a bit of heat.

1 cup finely shredded green cabbage

2 carrots, grated

1 green capsicum, seeded and thinly sliced

1 red capsicum, seeded and thinly sliced

1 small cucumber, grated

4 tablespoons of pure maple syrup, agave syrup or brown sugar

1 teaspoon of salt

3 tablespoons vegan fish sauce (or, if you can't find it, use vegetarian oyster sauce)

3 garlic cloves, crushed

2 tablespoons of lime juice

1 teaspoon vegetable stock powder

2 tablespoons of olive oil

300 g rice noodles

1 cup fresh basil leaves

¼ cup roasted peanuts

fried Asian shallots, for sprinkling

- Place the cabbage, carrots, capsicums and cucumber in a large bowl. Stir to combine, then set aside.

- In another bowl, make a dressing by whisking together the maple syrup, salt, vegan fish sauce (or soy sauce and extra lime juice), garlic, lime juice, stock powder and olive oil until well combined. Set aside.

- Cook the rice noodles following the packet instructions. Drain and refresh under cold running water, then drain again.

- Toss the noodles through the vegetable mixture. Pour the dressing over and gently mix it through.

- Just before serving, mix the basil leaves through. Garnish with the peanuts, sprinkle with the fried shallots and serve.

Recipe contributed by Melanie Baker, The Kind Cook

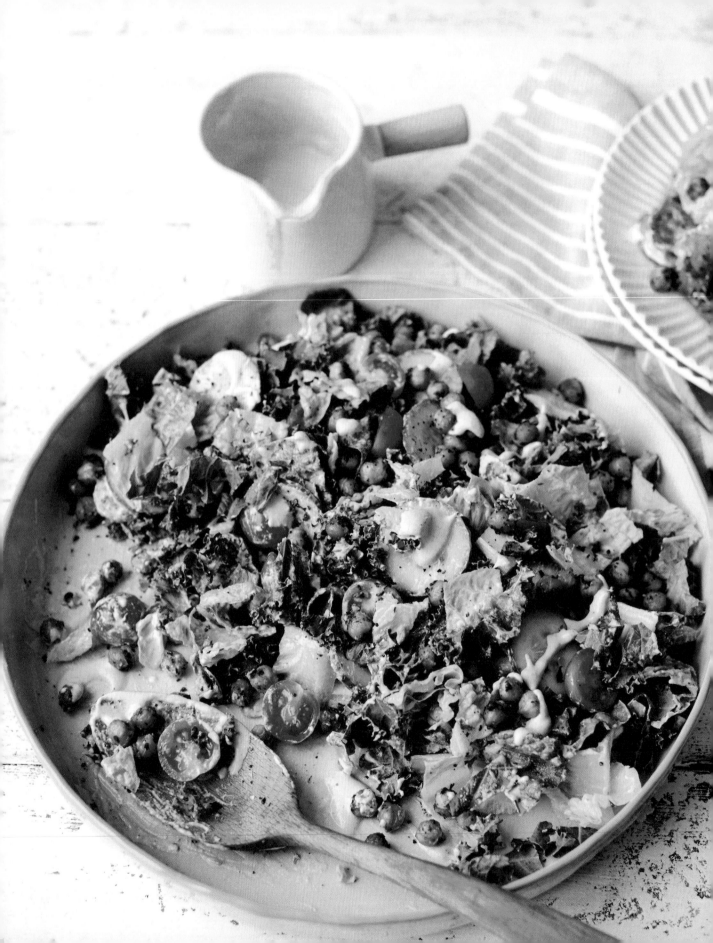

Caesar Salad with Herb-roasted Chickpeas

SERVES 4

Crunchy and fresh with a flavour-packed creamy dressing, this salad will make you excited about eating your greens. The secret ingredient in the dressing is aquafaba – a fancy name for the liquid from a tin of chickpeas. Here, this versatile ingredient is whipped to add a mayonnaise-like creaminess to the caesar dressing.

1 cos lettuce
1 bunch kale, stems removed
1 small Lebanese cucumber
1 punnet cherry tomatoes

HERB-ROASTED CHICKPEAS

400 g tin chickpeas, liquid reserved
1½ tablespoons virgin olive oil
1 tablespoon lemon juice
1 teaspoon dried basil
1 teaspoon dried parsley
1 teaspoon smoked paprika (optional)
1 teaspoon onion powder or granules
½ teaspoon fine sea salt
¼ teaspoon cracked black pepper,
  or to taste

CAESAR DRESSING

½ cup raw unsalted cashews, soaked
  for at least 10 minutes in boiling
  water, or overnight in cold water
1½ tablespoons aquafaba (the liquid
  from the tin of chickpeas)
1 tablespoon lemon juice
1½ teaspoons tamari or soy sauce
  (gluten-free, if needed)
1–2 garlic cloves, peeled
2 teaspoons dijon mustard
2 teaspoons capers, drained
½ teaspoon fine sea salt
¼ teaspoon cracked black pepper
3 tablespoons mild-flavoured olive
  oil or canola oil

- Preheat the oven to 175°C conventional, or 155°C fan-forced.

- To prepare the chickpeas, drain the tin of chickpeas, reserving the liquid for the salad dressing. Toss the chickpeas in a mixing bowl with the olive oil, lemon juice, dried herbs and spices. Pour into a large glass baking dish and roast for 25–35 minutes, or until the chickpeas are crunchy, stirring every 7–8 minutes so they colour evenly. Remove from the oven and leave to cool.

- Near serving time, place all the dressing ingredients, except the olive oil, in a blender. Add ⅓ cup water and blend on high until smooth. With the motor running, slowly drizzle the olive oil into the blender. Blend for about 1 minute, until all the ingredients are incorporated and the dressing is smooth and creamy. Taste test and add more salt and pepper as desired.

- Wash all the vegetables and dry them thoroughly. (Salad dressing won't stick to wet vegies and will pool at the bottom of your bowl instead of coating them evenly.) Chop the lettuce and kale into bite-sized pieces and place in a large salad bowl. Slice the cucumber into rounds, cut the cherry tomatoes and add to the salad bowl.

- Just before serving, drizzle the dressing over the salad and gently toss until all the vegetables are well coated. Top with the roasted chickpeas and watch this delicious salad disappear.

Scented Crunchy Black Rice Salad

SERVES 2

An aromatic salad, showcasing a range of fragrant Asian flavours. Nuts, noodles and coriander roots add a gorgeous crunch. For extra kick, simply leave the seeds in the chilli – or, if you're feeling brave, add more chilli!

½ cup black rice (you could try the glutinous version)

1–2 tablespoons vegetable oil

½ small brown onion, finely diced

10 mushrooms (preferably Asian, or you can use button mushrooms), sliced

⅓ cup well-washed, finely sliced coriander roots

a handful of coriander leaves, roughly chopped

a handful of basil leaves, torn

a handful of baby spinach leaves

1 small red chilli, cut in half lengthwise, seeds removed and finely sliced

a handful of crunchy fried Asian noodles

2 handfuls of peanuts, toasted (see tip)

SOY, LIME AND SESAME DRESSING

1 tablespoon soy sauce (or tamari, for a gluten-free option)

¼ teaspoon sesame oil

2 teaspoons lime juice

¼ teaspoon finely chopped fresh ginger

1 teaspoon pure maple syrup

1 large garlic clove, crushed

- Rinse the rice under cold water. Place it in a saucepan of water, bring to the boil, then reduce the heat and simmer for 30–40 minutes, or until the rice is tender. If you're using gelatinous rice, you might like to rinse it after it is cooked to remove any starches. Drain and set aside.

- While the rice is simmering, heat a good dash of the vegetable oil in a small frying pan and sauté the onion over medium heat for about 10 minutes, or until it caramelises. Add the mushrooms and cook for 5–10 minutes, until they are softened and coloured. Using tongs, remove the mixture from the pan and set aside on paper towel to drain.

- In a large bowl, whisk together all the dressing ingredients. Add the cooked rice, mushroom mixture, sliced coriander roots, herbs and spinach and toss together.

- Just before serving, sprinkle with the chilli, noodles and nuts, so they stay super crunchy.

- Serve warm or cold.

Tip
To toast raw peanuts, toss them in a hot frying pan for 1–2 minutes.

Recipe contributed by **Melanie Baker, The Kind Cook**

Potato, Kale and Pine Nut Salad

SERVES 6-8 AS A SIDE

Massages shouldn't be reserved for stressed-out office workers. By treating the kale in this salad with a little TLC, it will transform to emerald velvet in your hands, and work magic on your tastebuds. Combine with smashed potato, creamy mayo and pine nuts, pep it all up with a little spring onion herbage, and you'll have people gobbling down their greens in no time, no problem.

3 medium-large waxy or boiling
   potatoes, peeled and cut into
   2 cm cubes

2 large bunches curly kale

1 tablespoon olive oil

zest and juice of 1 lemon or lime

1 tablespoon unhulled tahini

4–6 spring onions, finely chopped,
   or ½ red onion, finely sliced

1 beetroot, peeled and grated

2–4 tablespoons agave syrup
   or maple syrup

1–2 tablespoons capers in
   brine, drained

1 small bunch basil, leaves picked
   and rinsed

2 tablespoons pine nuts, raw
   or toasted

Lemon-basil mayo (see page 157),
   for drizzling

- Bring a large saucepan of salted water to the boil. Carefully add the diced potatoes. Boil for about 10 minutes, or until the potatoes are tender, and just starting to fall apart. Some cubes will remain whole, while others will dissolve to help create a kind of dressing for the kale. Drain in a colander and set aside to cool.

- Thoroughly wash the kale, then strip the leaves off the tough central stems. Tear the leaves into bite-sized pieces and place in a large bowl. Add the olive oil, lemon zest, lemon juice and tahini. Sprinkle with a pinch of salt and pepper.

- Now, roll up your sleeves and get your hands in there! Give the kale a good squeeze to help tenderise it – the colour will change as you do this, turning a richer shade of green. Add the cooled potatoes, spring onions, beetroot, agave syrup, capers and most of the basil leaves, then give another quick toss.

- Tip the mixture into your serving bowl and scatter with the pine nuts and a few reserved basil leaves. Serve with the lemon-basil mayo for lucky diners to dollop on top, and you're done!

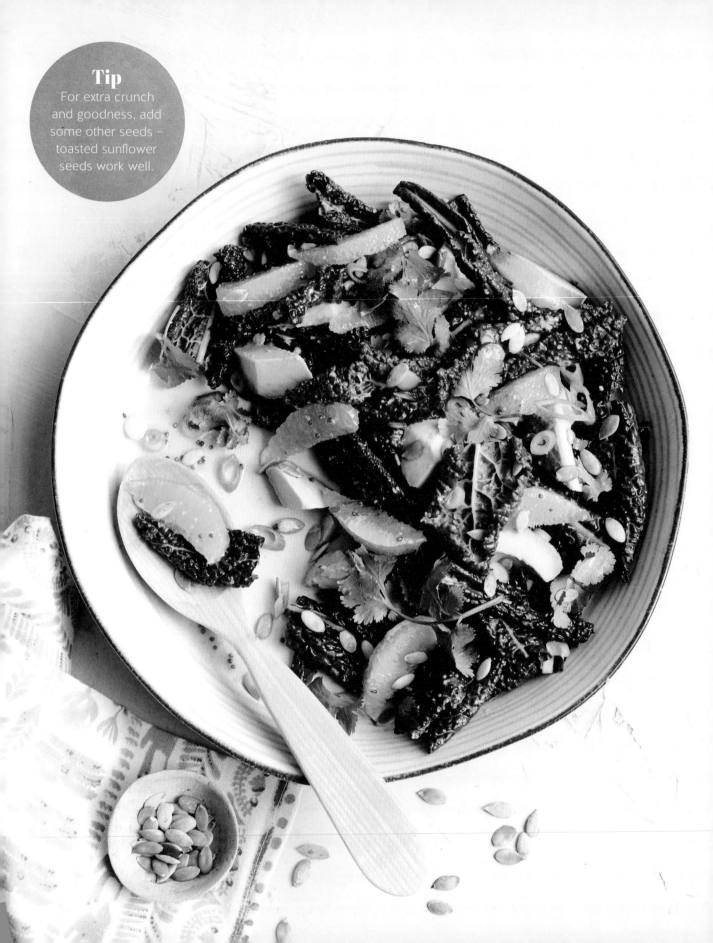

Tip
For extra crunch and goodness, add some other seeds – toasted sunflower seeds work well.

Tuscan Kale, Orange and Avocado Salad

SERVES 2-4

Crunchy kale and creamy avocado complement each other beautifully in this fresh, zesty salad. Kale will really sing in a salad if you give it a little bit of love! Rubbing salt into the leaves will not only remove any bitterness, but will turn the leaves a glossy green right before your eyes. We've used a mustard-based dressing here, but anything with a hint of sweetness will work well. This is a delightful salad on its own or as a side dish, and is a lovely way to enjoy kale. As kale doesn't wilt quickly, this salad will keep well in the fridge overnight.

½ cup pumpkin seeds
1 bunch Tuscan kale
sea salt, for sprinkling
1 orange, peeled and cut
    into bite-sized pieces
½ ripe avocado, cut into
    bite-sized pieces
1 cup finely chopped spring onions
1 cup finely chopped coriander leaves,
    plus extra leaves to garnish

LEMON DIJON DRESSING
juice of 1 small lemon or lime
2 tablespoons extra virgin olive oil
1 teaspoon dijon mustard
1 teaspoon agave syrup

- Toast the pumpkin seeds over low heat in a non-stick frying pan. Remove from the pan and set aside.

- In a bowl, whisk together all the dressing ingredients. Season to taste with salt and pepper and set aside.

- Wash the kale, then strip the leaves off the tough central stems. Roughly chop the leaves and sprinkle with the sea salt. Vigorously massage the salt into the leaves; you'll quickly see them turn a glossy, bright green.

- Place the kale in a serving bowl. Add the orange, avocado and spring onion and gently toss together. Sprinkle with the coriander and toasted pumpkin seeds, drizzle with the dressing and serve.

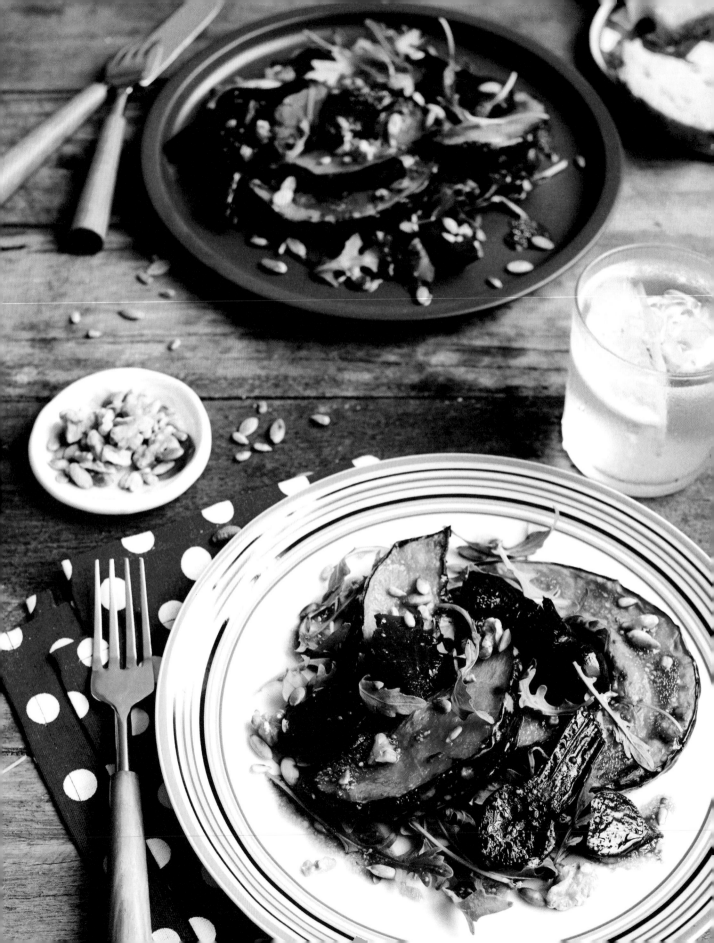

Roasted Beetroot and Pumpkin Salad with Rocket and Walnuts

SERVES 2-4

It's hard to decide what's the hero of this salad – the sweet and sticky mustard seed dressing, or the roasted vegies it clings to so deliciously. A peppery rocket base and generous mix of nuts and seeds make this elegant dish as healthy as it is tasty.

800 g kent pumpkin
1-2 tablespoons olive oil
1 bunch (about 6-8) baby beetroot
250 g rocket leaves
½ cup walnuts, lightly crushed
¼ cup sunflower seeds
¼ cup pumpkin seeds

SEEDED MUSTARD DRESSING

2 tablespoons extra virgin olive oil
2 teaspoons wholegrain mustard
2 teaspoons maple syrup or agave
   syrup syrup
2 teaspoons balsamic vinegar
2 teaspoons apple cider vinegar
½ teaspoon sesame oil

- Preheat the oven to 200°C conventional, or 180°C fan-forced. Line two baking trays with baking paper.
- Slice the pumpkin into thin wedges, leaving the skin on to help the wedges keep their shape. Toss with the olive oil and a pinch of salt and arrange on one of the baking trays.
- Wash the beetroot and slice the tops off. Wrap them individually in foil, then place on the other baking tray.
- Roast for about 30 minutes, or until you can easily poke a knife through the beetroot; the beetroot may take a little longer to cook than the pumpkin.
- Carefully unwrap the beetroot and rinse under cold water. The skins should slide right off, or you can leave them on. Cut each beetroot into halves or quarters and set aside to cool with the pumpkin.
- In a small bowl, whisk all the dressing ingredients together. Season with salt and pepper, then taste and add a little more maple syrup or vinegar if you think the dressing needs it.
- Put the rocket in a serving bowl and top with the cooled beetroot and pumpkin. Add the walnuts, sunflower seeds and pumpkin seeds. Drizzle with the dressing and serve immediately.

Tip

If you don't have time to roast your own beetroot, use the precooked beetroot sold vacuum-packed in the fruit and veg section of the supermarket.

Roasted Tomato, Artichoke and Bean Salad

SERVES 4-6

This isn't an old-fashioned wishy-washy limp-greens salad: it's substantial and rich in protein, thanks to the addition of butterbeans and chickpeas, while roasting the tomatoes brings out all their natural sweetness, and creates a light sauce that coats simply blanched green beans and tender artichoke hearts. This salad also travels fabulously well, so it's great for packing into picnic baskets or lunchboxes. Serve with crusty bread to soak up all the juices.

500 g (2 punnets) cherry tomatoes

2 small red onions, cut into
thin wedges

1 red capsicum, seeded and cut into
1 cm slices

400 g tin artichoke hearts in brine
(not marinated in oil)

2 tablespoons olive oil

a generous pinch of sea salt

400 g green beans, trimmed

400 g tin butterbeans, drained
but not rinsed

400 g tin chickpeas, drained but
not rinsed

⅓ cup roughly chopped parsley

lemon wedges, to serve

TAHINI-TARRAGON VINAIGRETTE

juice of 1 lemon

2 teaspoons olive oil

2 teaspoons dijon mustard

2 teaspoons unhulled tahini

1 teaspoon aged balsamic vinegar

1 small French shallot, finely diced

- Preheat the oven to 220°C conventional, or 200°C fan-forced. Line a large baking tray with baking paper.

- Wash and dry the cherry tomatoes, then spread them over the baking tray. Scatter with the onion and capsicum. Drain the artichoke hearts, cut them in half and place, cut side up, on the baking tray. Drizzle the whole lot with the olive oil, and sprinkle with the salt, then roast for 20 minutes, or until the vegetables are starting to char ever so slightly, and some tomatoes have split to release their juices. Remove from the oven and allow to cool.

- Meanwhile, drop the green beans into a large saucepan of boiling salted water and blanch for 2 minutes. Drain, then quickly plunge into a bowl or sink full of iced water, to preserve their colour. Drain in a colander, then pat dry with a clean tea towel.

- Toss the green beans into a large bowl. Add the butterbeans, chickpeas, parsley and roasted vegetables – including any of the roasting juices left on the baking tray. Gently mix so that some tomatoes burst and coat the beans, and some remain more or less whole. Season with pepper, then tip the whole lot into a large serving dish.

- Combine all the vinaigrette ingredients in a clean airtight jar, close the lid tightly and shake vigorously. Pour into a small jug and serve alongside the salad, for diners to help themselves. Serve with lemon wedges, for squeezing over.

Tip

For a more substantial salad, add some quartered, boiled potatoes.

Creamy Apple, Beetroot and Carrot Salad

SERVES 4

There are certain recipes that redefine what a salad can be, and this is one of them. At the heart of this colourful salad is the 'ABC' trio of apple, beetroot and carrot. It's fresh, filling and flavoursome! And did we mention it's pink? If you want to mix it up, try adding leafy greens, tomato and celery. And if you'd like your salad very creamy, you can always make more dressing.

1 green apple
1 beetroot
2 carrots
1 tablespoon sesame seeds
1 tablespoon pumpkin seeds
1 tablespoon currants

CREAMY CASHEW DRESSING
¼ cup cashews
⅓ cup soy milk, or other
   dairy-free milk
1 garlic clove
juice of 1 lemon
2 teaspoons olive oil
½ teaspoon dijon or
   wholegrain mustard
½ teaspoon salt

- Peel and grate the apple, beetroot and carrot. Place in a bowl with the sesame seeds, pumpkin seeds and currants and toss together.
- Place all the dressing ingredients in a blender or food processor and blend until smooth.
- Pour the dressing over the salad. Toss together and serve.

Tip
For a super smooth dressing, pre-soak raw cashews overnight.

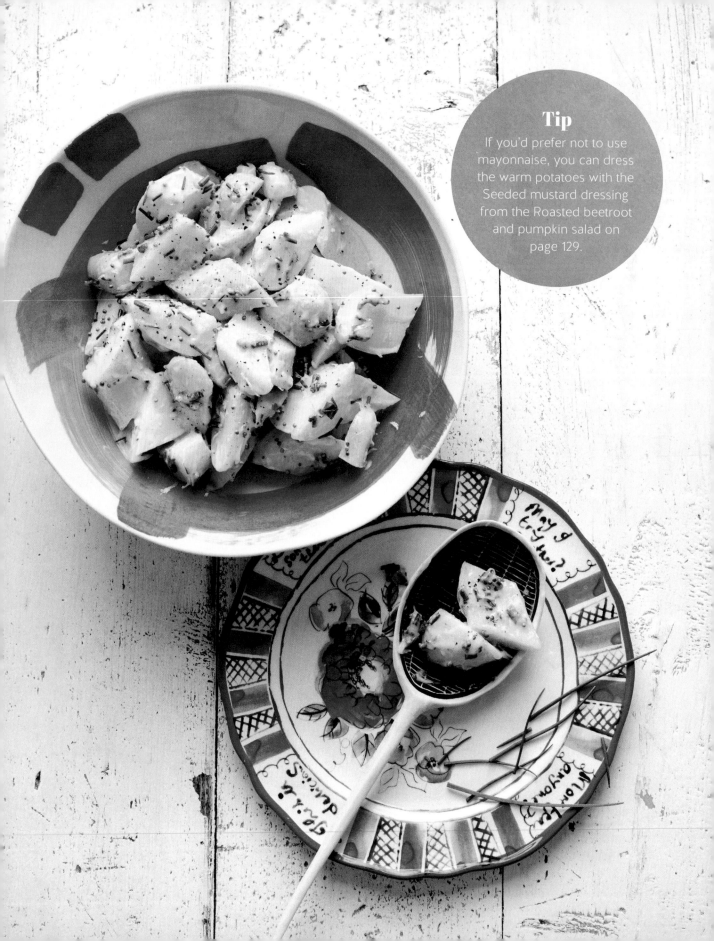

Tip

If you'd prefer not to use mayonnaise, you can dress the warm potatoes with the Seeded mustard dressing from the Roasted beetroot and pumpkin salad on page 129.

Classic Potato Salad

SERVES 4

This zesty summer salad is perfect at a backyard barbie to accompany some grilled vegie snags or mushrooms. 'New' potatoes make the tastiest potato salads due to their sweetness and buttery texture. There is no need to peel them as the skins are so thin.

500 g new season waxy potatoes, such as golden delight, nicola or kipfler
½ teaspoon yellow or brown mustard seeds
½ cup egg-free mayonnaise (see tip)
½ teaspoon dijon mustard
1 teaspoon apple cider vinegar
1 teaspoon finely grated lemon zest
a handful of finely chopped chives

- Wash the potatoes and place them whole in a saucepan of cold water. Bring to the boil, then reduce the heat and simmer for about 20 minutes, or until a knife can slide easily into the potatoes. Don't overcook them though – you don't want them falling apart when you drain them.
- While the potatoes are simmering, heat a frying pan over medium heat. Add the mustard seeds to the dry pan and toast for about 30 seconds, until they smell aromatic and begin to pop, keeping an eye on them so they don't burn. Take them off the heat straight away.
- In a small bowl, whisk together the mayonnaise, mustard, vinegar, lemon zest and a pinch of salt until smooth. Stir in the chives and mustard seeds.
- When the potatoes are tender, drain them and leave for 10–15 minutes to cool to room temperature.
- Cut the cooled potatoes into halves or quarters, depending on how big you'd like them. Place in a salad bowl and mix gently with the dressing. Serve immediately, or cover and pop in the fridge to serve chilled later.

Variations

- Add 1 large crushed garlic clove to the dressing, if desired.
- For a sweet flavour, add raw fresh corn kernels or grated carrot.
- For a bit of crunch, add chopped celery or sliced Lebanese cucumber.
- A tablespoon or so of chopped fresh dill is also delicious and creates a pickle flavour.

Quinoa Tabouleh

SERVES 6

~~~~~~~~

This fresh Middle Eastern-inspired salad is perfect for wraps or as a side, and always shines with its old friends hummus and falafel. Tabouleh is traditionally made with cracked wheat, but this version uses protein-packed quinoa, making it a little more filling. For some extra Omega-3 and Omega-6, you could also replace some of the olive oil with flaxseed oil.

1 red onion, finely diced
3 garlic cloves, crushed
juice of 3 lemons
⅓ cup olive oil
1 teaspoon salt
⅓ cup quinoa
2 Lebanese cucumbers, peeled and diced
4 tomatoes, diced
1 bunch parsley, finely chopped

- In a bowl, mix together the onion, garlic, lemon juice, olive oil, salt and some pepper to taste. Set aside.

- Rinse the quinoa thoroughly, then place in a small saucepan with ⅔ cup water. Bring to the boil, then reduce the heat, put the lid on and leave to simmer for about 10 minutes, or until all the water has been absorbed. Set aside to cool.

- Combine the cucumber, tomato and parsley in a large salad bowl. Add the quinoa, then pour the onion mixture over the salad.

- Toss everything together and you're ready to serve. This salad is best enjoyed the day it is made.

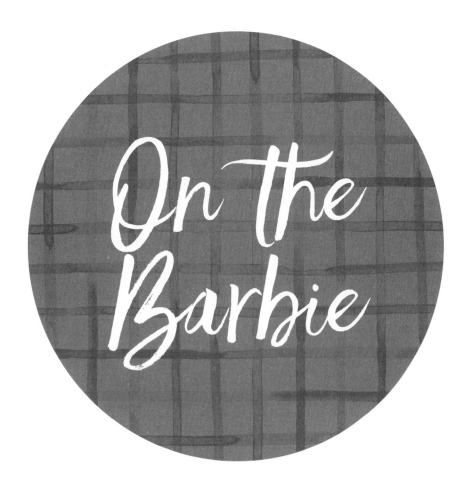

On the Barbie

Basically, when meat-free patties, snags or vegies meet the hotplate, *magic happens*. Not convinced? You will be once you experience tempting satay kebabs, black bean burgers and miso-glazed eggplant.

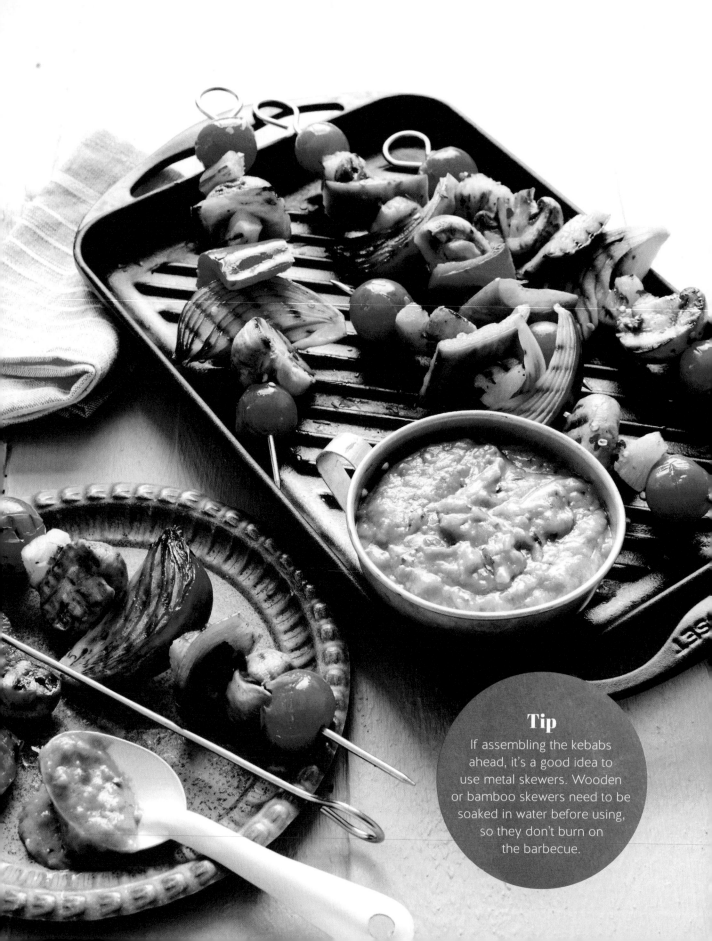

Tip

If assembling the kebabs
ahead, it's a good idea to
use metal skewers. Wooden
or bamboo skewers need to be
soaked in water before using,
so they don't burn on
the barbecue.

Vegetable Kebabs with Satay Sauce

MAKES 8 SKEWERS; SERVES 4

Sweet satay is a nutty and delectable sauce for these crisp and colourful vegie kebabs, which make a healthy and tasty addition to any summer barbecue. You can easily assemble the kebabs at home, then just take them along to a barbecue to share around with friends or family.

2 red onions
24 button mushrooms
2 red and/or green capsicums
500 g (2 punnets) cherry tomatoes
2 x 225 g tins pineapple chunks

SATAY SAUCE
1 tablespoon coconut oil
1 small brown onion, finely diced
1 tablespoon grated fresh ginger
1 garlic clove, crushed
1 tablespoon finely chopped
    coriander leaves
2 tablespoons finely chopped
    fresh lemongrass
2 tablespoons crunchy peanut butter
1 tablespoon grated palm sugar
2 tablespoons soy sauce
1 tablespoon sweet chilli sauce
1 tablespoon lime or lemon juice
270 ml coconut cream

- If using wooden or bamboo skewers, soak them in cold water for an hour before using, so they don't burn on the barbecue.

- Chop the onion, mushrooms and capsicum into bite-sized chunks, about an inch wide.

- Thread a whole cherry tomato onto each skewer by piercing it through the middle, leaving a few inches free at the bottom of the skewer for easy handling during cooking and eating. Alternate a piece of each vegetable and the pineapple onto each skewer, ending with another cherry tomato to keep everything in place, and leaving about an inch of skewer free at the top.

- To make the satay sauce, melt the coconut oil in a saucepan and fry the onion, ginger, garlic, coriander and lemongrass over medium heat for about 5 minutes, until the onion starts to brown.

- Stir in the peanut butter, until it has melted, then stir in the palm sugar, soy sauce, sweet chilli sauce and lime juice.

- Now add the coconut cream, mixing constantly and scraping the bottom of the pan to make sure all the ingredients are well combined. Keep cooking and stirring for about 3 minutes until you see a few bubbles, then immediately remove from the heat, so the coconut cream doesn't separate. Keep stirring for a few moments. (If taking to a barbecue, store in an airtight container and gently reheat before serving.)

- When ready to cook the kebabs, preheat the barbecue to medium–high. Add the skewers and cook for 5 minutes on both sides, or until the vegetables are well grilled but not overcooked, or they may start to fall off the skewer.

- Cover generously with the satay sauce and serve.

Beasty Black Bean Burger Patties

MAKES 8 PATTIES

This burger patty wants to be the centre of attention. It's not only hearty and filling, but also packs a serious flavour punch. It goes well with any classic burger fillings, and exceptionally well with egg-free mayo or aioli. Check out pages 182–7 for a great range of dairy-free cheeses you can also add to your burger.

vegetable oil, for pan-frying

scant ⅔ cup chickpea flour (besan) or plain flour

2 teaspoons baking powder

2 x 400 g tins black beans, rinsed and drained

⅓ cup olive oil

⅓ cup red wine

1 tablespoon soy sauce

2 teaspoons balsamic vinegar

1 teaspoon salt

1 teaspoon black pepper

1 teaspoon ground dried sage

a pinch of dried rosemary

• Preheat a barbecue hotplate to medium-low. Brush with vegetable oil. (Alternatively, you can use a large frying pan.)

• Set aside the flour, baking powder and half the black beans. Place all the other ingredients in a blender or food processor and blend for a few seconds.

• Tip the mixture into a bowl and mix through the second tin of black beans, the flour and baking powder.

• Shape the mixture into 8 patties, about 5 mm thick and 8 cm in diameter. Working in batches, cook the patties on the first side for 5–10 minutes, or until the bottom has begun to firm up, then flip them over and cook the other side for a further 5–10 minutes, or until browned and firm on each side.

• Serve hot, with your choice of burger toppings and fillings. These patties can also be served as a meal, with a side salad.

Sticky BBQ Tofu

SERVES 4 WITH RICE AND SALAD

This recipe makes tofu sing! The combination of flavours in the simple marinade work together to create a sticky-coated salty and sweet tofu that will spice up any dish.

¼ cup fermented black soy beans (see tip)

600 g firm tofu

2 tablespoons vegetable oil

1 small brown onion, finely diced

3 cm piece fresh ginger, peeled and grated

3 garlic cloves, crushed

1 small red chilli, finely chopped

1 teaspoon Chinese five-spice powder

1 cup vegetable stock

¼ cup soy sauce

1½ tablespoons apple cider vinegar

2 teaspoons sesame oil

⅓ cup brown sugar

4 prunes, pitted and chopped

1½ teaspoons cornflour, dissolved in 1 tablespoon water (optional)

- Soak the black soy beans in water for 1 hour, then rinse and drain. Mash them using a fork and set aside.

- Cut the tofu into slices about the width of a finger, then place on paper towel to dry a little.

- Meanwhile, make the marinade. In a small saucepan, heat the vegetable oil over medium heat. Add the onion, ginger, garlic and chilli and cook for about a minute, then add the five-spice and stir for a few minutes.

- Now stir in the mashed black soy beans and cook for another minute. Pour in the stock, soy sauce, vinegar and sesame oil, then stir in the sugar and prunes. Bring to the boil, reduce the heat to low and simmer, uncovered, for 10–12 minutes, or until the liquid has reduced by half. If the sauce needs thickening, stir in the cornflour mixture and simmer for another minute or so. Remove from the heat and leave to cool slightly. Using a stick blender, whiz until the marinade is smooth and glossy.

- Transfer to a bowl or airtight container, add the tofu and turn to coat all over. Cover and marinate in the fridge overnight.

- The next day, heat the barbecue to high. Drain the marinade into a small saucepan and warm it on the barbecue until heated through. Sear the tofu on the flat plate of the barbecue for about 2 minutes on each side, then transfer to a serving plate and drizzle with the hot, sticky marinade.

- Serve hot; it is especially delicious with the Fragrant Cambodian noodle salad on page 121.

Variation

- Instead of barbecuing the tofu, you could bake it. Simply put the tofu strips in a 25 cm x 35 cm baking dish, drizzle with the marinade and gently toss until coated. Bake in a preheated oven at 150°C conventional, or 130°C fan-forced, for 45–55 minutes, until the sauce is caramelised and sticky.

Tip

Fermented black soy beans, also known as 'douchi', provide the rich flavour base to this recipe. You'll find them in Asian grocery stores.

Recipe contributed by Suzy Spoon

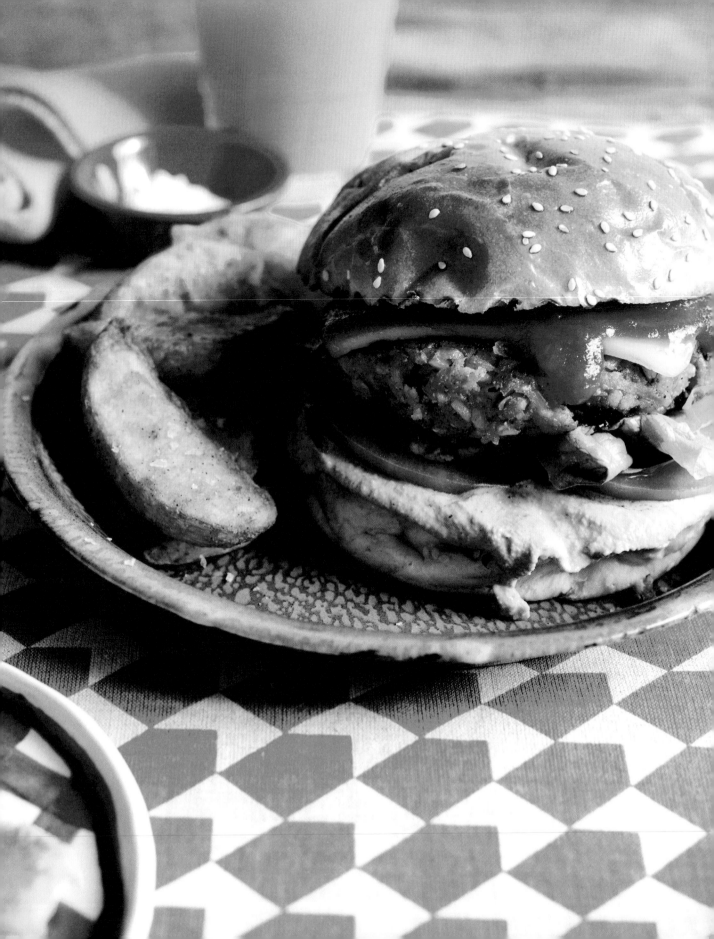

Sage and Onion Rissoles

MAKES 10-12 RISSOLES

Grilling these traditional English-style seasoned patties on the barbecue will give them a smoky hit that goes down a treat with potatoes, steamed greens or salad, and lashings of tomato sauce. Or, if it's the middle of winter and you don't feel like firing up the barbie, pan-fry them in a little olive oil over medium heat for about 5 minutes on each side, and you'll be rewarded with a lovely crispy crust on these little beauties.

2 cups cooked brown rice, cooled

1–1½ cups chopped mixed herbs
(parsley is a must; basil and
chives work well, too)

½–1½ cups panko breadcrumbs
(large Japanese ones)

400 g firm tofu, crumbled

1 large red onion, finely diced

1 carrot, grated

3–4 garlic cloves, crushed

2–3 tablespoons soy sauce
or tamari

2 tablespoons vegan
Worcestershire sauce

2 tablespoons olive oil

2 teaspoons sesame oil

2 tablespoons cornflour

1–2 tablespoons tomato paste

1 teaspoon sugar

2 teaspoons dried sage, crumbled

1 teaspoon onion powder

1 teaspoon garlic powder

½ teaspoon black pepper

¼ teaspoon ground allspice

rice bran or grapeseed oil,
for cooking

• Set aside the cooked cooled rice, chopped fresh herbs and breadcrumbs.

• Put all the remaining ingredients, except the vegetable oil, in a large bowl. Combine well, using your hands.

• Add the rice and chopped herbs and mix everything together. Gradually work in enough breadcrumbs to bind the mixture together – as you squash out the air, and the proteins start to bind, the mixture will take on a rissole texture. Cover the bowl and leave in the fridge for at least 5 minutes, or until you're ready to cook.

• Heat the flat plate of your barbecue to medium for at least 10 minutes. When it's hot, brush each rissole with a little oil and gently place on the hotplate. It's tempting to move them around, but just stand back and let them develop a nice, golden-brown crust. After about 5 minutes, have a peek underneath to make sure they're not burning. When they're golden underneath, carefully flip the rissoles over and brown the other side for a further 5–7 minutes, then you're all done.

Variation

• Try cooking the rice with vegan beef-style stock for extra flavour.

• For an extra protein power boost, use cooked and cooled quinoa in place of the brown rice.

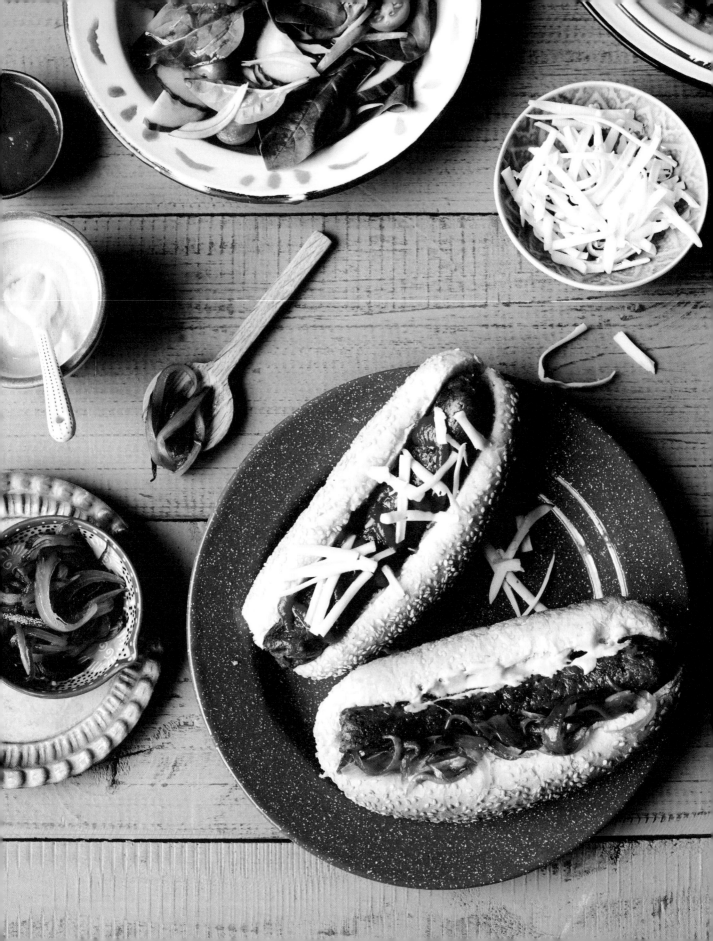

Spicy Italian Sausages

MAKES 6

Don't be overwhelmed by the thought of making your own sausages – these little guys are really straightforward to put together. The best thing you can give them, however, is time: chilling them in the fridge for a few hours will help ensure they hold together well on the barbie.

1 tablespoon ground flaxseeds
1 tablespoon olive oil
¼ cup finely chopped onion
1 cup finely chopped mushrooms
1 garlic clove, crushed
425 g tin black-eyed beans, rinsed
    and drained
2 tablespoons roughly chopped
    sundried tomatoes
2 tablespoons roughly chopped basil
¼ cup nutritional yeast
½ cup rice flour
3 tablespoons vegan Worcestershire
    sauce or soy sauce

CHILLI PAPRIKA SPICE MIX

1½ teaspoons garlic powder
½ teaspoon dried basil
½ teaspoon black pepper
1 teaspoon salt
1½ teaspoons sweet paprika
½ teaspoon smoked paprika
½ teaspoon chilli flakes
1 teaspoon dried oregano

- Put all the chilli paprika spice mix ingredients in a small bowl. Mix until well combined, then set aside.

- In another small bowl, mix the ground flaxseeds with 2½ tablespoons water and set aside to thicken. (This is known as a 'flax egg', and is used in egg-free cooking to help bind ingredients together.)

- Heat a frying pan over medium heat. Add 2 teaspoons of the olive oil and sauté the onion, mushrooms and garlic for about 5 minutes, or until softened. Set aside to cool.

- Put the black-eyed beans in a large bowl. Using a potato masher or your hands, mash them up a little to break the beans apart. (You can use a food processor, but be careful not to make a purée – you want the beans to have lots of texture.)

- Add the sundried tomatoes, basil, nutritional yeast, rice flour and the chilli paprika spice mix and mix together well. Add the flaxseed mixture and mix well until combined, then add the cooled vegetable mixture, Worcestershire or soy sauce and remaining of oil. Mix again until well combined.

- Bring a large saucepan of water to the boil. Set aside six pieces of foil, to wrap your sausages in.

- Divide the sausage mixture into six even portions. To shape your sausages, roll them gently between your hands. They will take more shape if you then put them on the foil sheets and roll them gently, as if you're rolling out play-dough. You can mould the ends of the foil-wrapped sausage with your hands to get a nice rounded shape. Roll them up in the foil, then secure the ends, like Christmas bon-bons.

- Place the sausages in a metal steamer, on top of the saucepan of boiling water. Cover and steam for 15–20 minutes.

- Remove from the heat and allow to cool, leaving them in their foil wrapping. Refrigerate the sausages for a few hours, or overnight if possible, to help them firm up.

- When you're ready to sizzle, unwrap the sausages and cook them on a hot barbecue over medium heat for about 10 minutes, or until heated through and nicely browned all over, taking care when turning the sausages as they are quite fragile. Serve warm.

Recipe contributed by Rhea Parsons

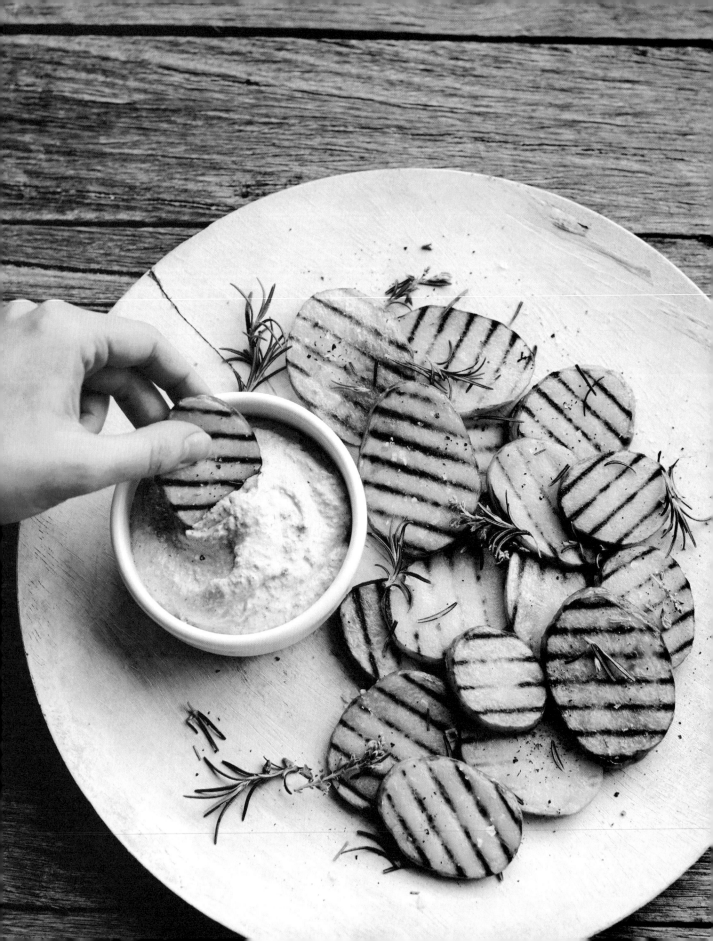

Grilled Potato Slices with Herbed Sour Cream

SERVES 4

Potatoes, rosemary, olive oil and salt. What more is there to say?

4 large, waxy potatoes
½ cup olive oil, approximately
3 garlic cloves, sliced
2 tablespoons finely chopped
　　rosemary
2 teaspoons salt

HERBED SOUR CREAM
1–1½ cups Cashew sour cream
　　(page 159)
½ cup basil leaves
1 spring onion, roughly chopped

- Scrub the potatoes well, but don't peel them. Cut into slices 1 cm thick, place in a large saucepan and pour in enough cold water to just cover them. Bring to the boil then reduce the heat to a simmer and cook for about 4 minutes, or until the potatoes are just tender – don't let them fall apart! Drain carefully through a colander, then leave to dry out for at least 10 minutes.

- Meanwhile, put the herbed sour cream ingredients in a blender, season with pepper and whiz until bright green and gorgeous. Set aside in a small serving bowl.

- In a wide shallow dish, mix together the olive oil, garlic, rosemary and salt. Add your air-dried potato slices and leave for a few minutes to soak up some of the garlicky oil.

- Heat the flat plate of your barbecue to high. Cook your potato slices until golden – about 5–7 minutes on each side should do it.

- Carefully transfer to a serving plate, then season with salt and pepper to taste. Serve hot, with the herbed sour cream on the side as a dipping sauce.

Tip
For a chargrilled effect, you can cook the potato slices on the open grill of your barbecue if you're feeling brave! Or you can use a chargrill pan inside.

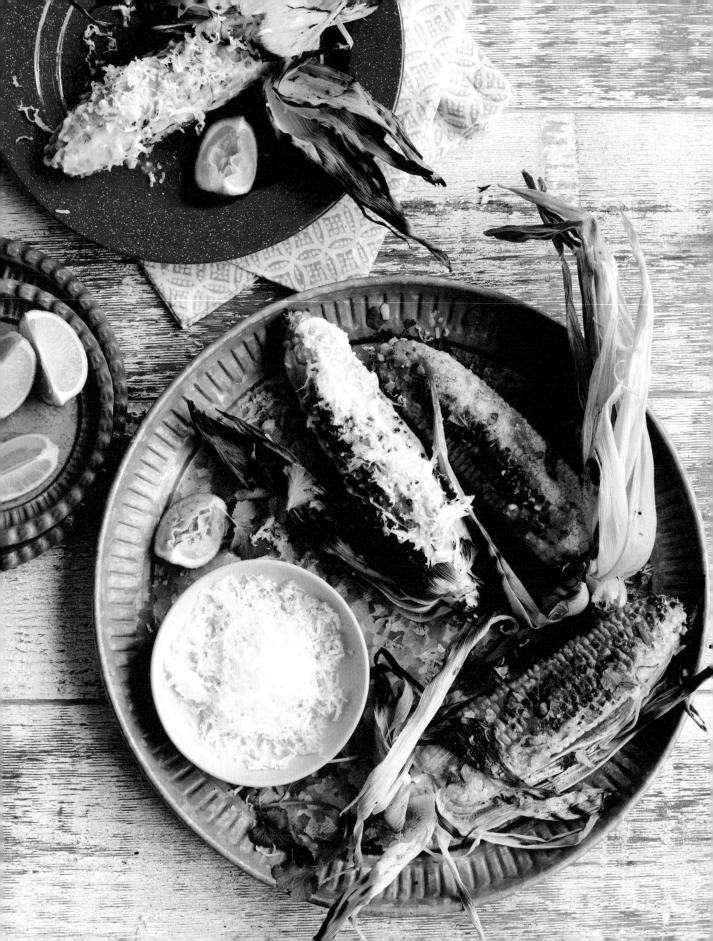

Grilled Corn 2 Ways

SERVES 4

The freshest corn + barbecue = simple perfection. The only question is to shuck or not to shuck? Leaving the husks on can make eating a little messy, but your corn will be bursting with juicy goodness. Grilling the corn 'naked' will give you a lovely charred flavour, but the kernels will be slightly less juicy. The choice is yours. It's easy to whip up a huge pile of these cobs for a Mexican-themed party. Also, check out the Spicy bean nachos on page 172.

4 corn cobs
1 lime, cut into wedges

SPICED LIME AND CORIANDER CORN

⅓ cup melted coconut oil
2 teaspoons sweet paprika (or smoked paprika, if you'd like an extra smoky barbecue hit!)
a pinch of cayenne pepper (optional)
1 small bunch coriander, chopped

ELOTES (MEXICAN STREET-STYLE CORN)

⅓ cup melted coconut oil or dairy-free margarine
¼ cup egg-free mayonnaise
¼–½ cup finely grated dairy-free cheese (see tip)

- Heat your barbecue to medium–high.

- Remove the husks and silks from the corn, if desired. Place the cobs on the barbecue and cook, turning often, for 7–10 minutes, until the corn turns a deep golden colour, with a few charred patches.

- If you're cooking your cobs with the husks on, lightly char them on the barbecue for 7–10 minutes, turning frequently, until nicely browned all over.

- For the spiced lime and coriander corn, brush the cooked cobs with the melted coconut oil, then sprinkle with the paprika, a pinch of salt and pepper, and the cayenne pepper, if using. Scatter the chopped coriander over and serve with lime wedges.

- For the elotes, roll the cooked cobs in the melted coconut oil, then in the mayonnaise. Sprinkle with the cheese, and salt and pepper if desired. Serve with lime wedges.

Tip

See pages 182–7 for some dairy-free cheeses you can make yourself.

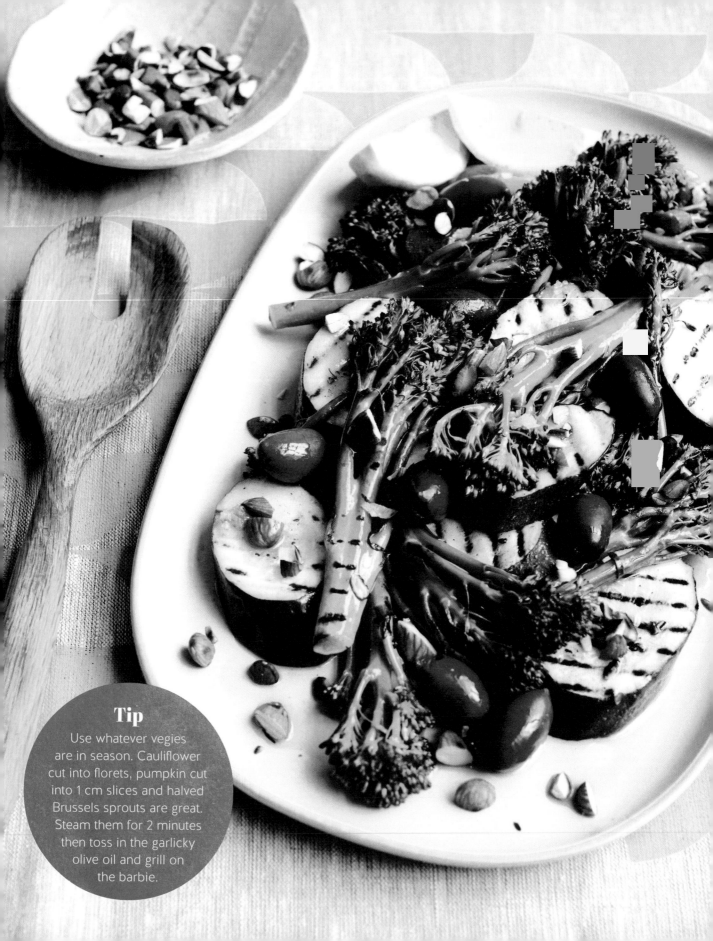

Tip

Use whatever vegies are in season. Cauliflower cut into florets, pumpkin cut into 1 cm slices and halved Brussels sprouts are great. Steam them for 2 minutes then toss in the garlicky olive oil and grill on the barbie.

Barbecued Vegie Plate with Almonds and Olives

SERVES 4

Break out of the box by grilling your greens instead of boiling them. Add some Grilled potato slices (page 147), Mexican street-style corn (page 149), a kale salad with Lemon-basil mayo (page 157), a few big jugs of frozen margaritas and a few great friends and, oh boy, you've got yourself the recipe for a perfect summer weekend.

3 bunches broccolini (about 15 stems)
2 large zucchini, cut into thick slices
3–4 tablespoons olive oil
1 garlic clove, crushed
150–200 g unpitted kalamata olives
100 g raw almonds
lemon wedges, to serve

- Heat your barbecue to medium–high.

- In a double-boiler or microwave, lightly steam the broccolini for 1–1½ minutes, or until bright green and just tender. Immediately blanch in iced water to stop the cooking process, then drain well and place in a large bowl.

- Zucchini doesn't need precooking, so just add it straight to the bowl. Drizzle with the olive oil, add the garlic and season with salt and pepper to taste. Toss gently.

- When you're ready to cook, remove the broccolini and zucchini using tongs, letting the excess oil drip back into the bowl, and place on the grill plate of your barbecue. Quickly toss the olives and almonds in the leftover garlic oil mixture, then place on the flat plate of your barbecue.

- Grill the broccolini and zucchini for a few minutes on each side, until lightly charred, and cook the olives and almonds for a few minutes, until warmed through.

- Transfer the grilled greens to a warmed serving plate. Scatter the warm olives and almonds over and serve with lemon wedges.

Grilled Mushrooms 2 Ways

SERVES 4

Do you want to know the secret to perfectly grilled mushrooms? Marinate them after you've seared them on the barbecue – that way they'll soak up all the seasonings for maximum juiciness, without burning. Use the best balsamic vinegar you can afford. Generally graded on the label by a number of vine leaf symbols, 'four leaf' balsamic vinegar should have a sweet complexity that only comes with age, and you'll need just a little to season a dish to perfection.

4 large field mushrooms
¼ cup olive oil
green salad, to serve
crusty bread, to serve

BALSAMIC AND ONION MARINADE

2 teaspoons olive oil
1 small red onion, thinly sliced
   into half-moons
2–4 tablespoons aged balsamic
   vinegar
1 garlic clove, crushed (optional)
1 tablespoon chopped parsley
   or basil (optional)

WORCESTERSHIRE AND TAMARI GLAZE

2 teaspoons olive oil
2–4 tablespoons vegan
   Worcestershire sauce
2–4 tablespoons tamari
1 garlic clove, crushed (optional)
1 tablespoon chopped parsley
   or chives (optional)

- Preheat the barbecue to medium.
- Place all the balsamic and onion marinade ingredients, except the parsley or basil, in a bowl. Add a pinch of salt and pepper, whisk together and set aside.
- In a separate bowl, whisk together all the Worcestershire and tamari glaze ingredients, except the parsley or chives; add a pinch of pepper and set aside.
- Using a damp cloth, wipe any dirt from the mushrooms. Very carefully remove their stems. If the caps are very thick, make a small 'X' incision, or several shallow cuts, across the thickest section, being very careful not to cut all the way through. Brush the olive oil over all the mushrooms.
- Place the mushrooms, gill side down, on the hot barbecue grill plate and grill for 1–2 minutes, or until you get some faint grill marks. (By cooking this side first, all the lovely juices will remain inside the caps when you flip the mushrooms over, rather than falling onto the barbecue.) During cooking, brush with a little more olive oil if the mushrooms are looking a bit dry.
- Flip the mushrooms over and continue grilling until fork tender; this should take about 7–10 minutes, depending on their size.
- Place 2 of the hot mushrooms in the balsamic marinade, and the other 2 in the Worcestershire glaze, and let them soak for a minute or so.
- Sprinkle the reserved parsley or basil over the balsamic-marinated mushrooms, and the reserved parsley or chives over the others. Serve with a crisp green side salad, and lots of crusty bread to soak up all those lovely juices.

Variation

- Infuse a little Polish flavour into your mushrooms with a dill and garlic marinade, made by whisking 2 tablespoons olive oil together with 1–2 teaspoons dried dill, ½–¾ teaspoon salt, ½–¾ teaspoon garlic powder and a generous pinch of black pepper. Delicious with boiled baby potatoes, steamed broccoli and sauerkraut!

Miso-glazed Grilled Eggplant

SERVES 4 AS A SIDE

Eggplant with miso, or nasu dengaku, is a classic grilled Japanese dish. Once cooked, the sweet and salty glazed eggplant will separate easily from the skin when coaxed with a fork or chopsticks – although you can certainly devour the skin as well. This simple dish makes a delicious addition to just about any meal, but is lovely with a vegan miso soup and some steamed rice on the side.

2 large eggplants
salt, for sprinkling
2 tablespoons white miso paste
  (shiro miso)
1 tablespoon mirin
1 tablespoon sugar
1 tablespoon sesame oil
1 teaspoon sesame seeds
1 tablespoon chopped spring onion

- Using a sharp knife, cut the eggplants in half lengthways. On the inside surface of the halved eggplants, on the diagonal, cut 4–5 evenly spaced incisions, about 1–2 cm deep. Cut 4–5 more incisions in the opposite direction, to create a cubed effect.

- Sprinkle some salt on the eggplants and set aside for about 5 minutes, to let them release some of their juices and tenderise them.

- In a small bowl, combine the miso paste, mirin and sugar. Add 1 tablespoon water and whisk until smooth. Brush the miso glaze on the cut side of the eggplants, and into the incisions, reserving some glaze to baste with during cooking.

- Heat a chargrill pan or barbecue to medium. Add the sesame oil and allow to heat through. Add the eggplants, cut side down, and cook for about 10 minutes, until lightly browned and soft. Turn the eggplants over and cook for 3–4 minutes on the other side, brushing more glaze over the cut side. Flip again and cook on the cut side for another 3–4 minutes, until the glaze is caramelised.

- Serve warm, sprinkled with sesame seeds and spring onion.

Tip

Instead of grilling the glazed eggplants, you could roast them in a preheated oven at 200°C conventional, or 180°C fan-forced, for 20 minutes.

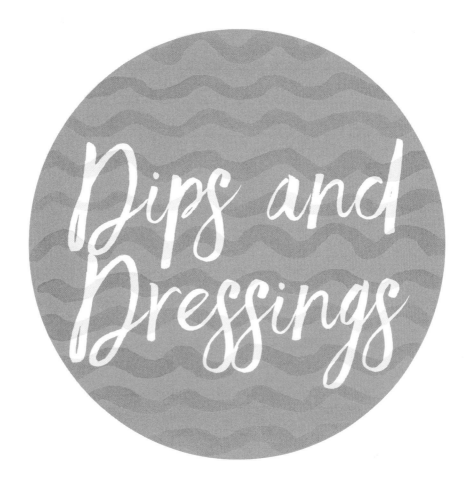

Dips and Dressings

A good condiment can elevate a 'meh' meal into something truly memorable. This selection is just the tip of a gigantic iceberg, from butter bean and basil dip to rich tzatziki and a guacamole that packs a punch.

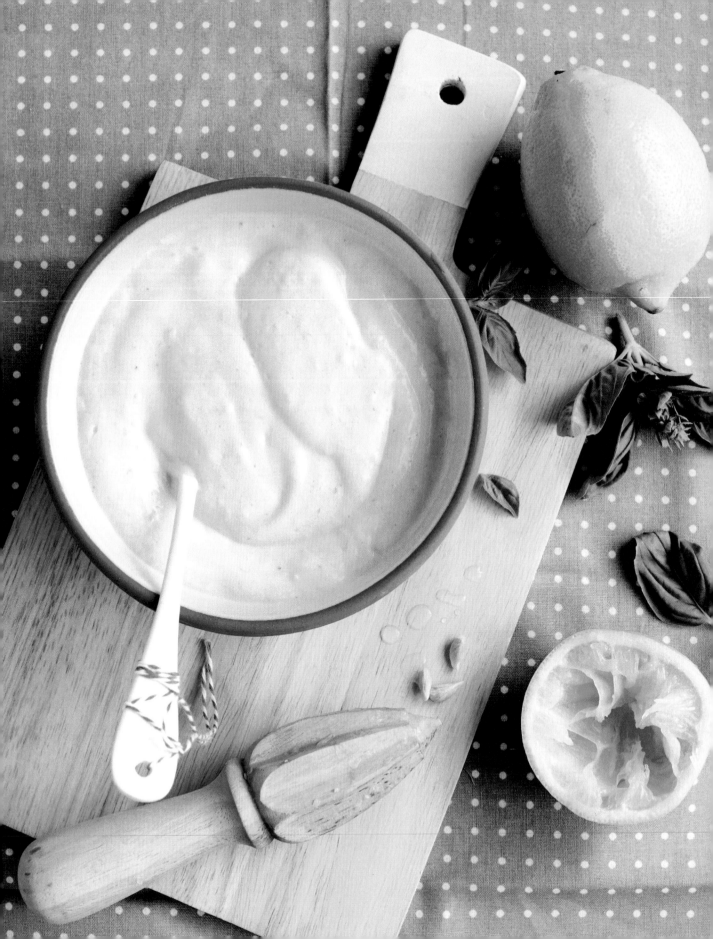

Lemon-basil Mayo

MAKES ABOUT 1½ CUPS

Fluffy, creamy and perfect for dips, dressings or dolloping, this mayo is egg free, cholesterol free and, best of all, animal friendly. It's adaptable, too: you can easily replace the basil with other herbs to suit the dish you're serving it with. Dill and coriander work particularly well.

300 g silken tofu
1 garlic clove, peeled
2–3 teaspoons sweet white miso
    paste (shiro miso)
zest and juice of 1 lemon
1 teaspoon sugar cane syrup (see tip)
2 teaspoons mild-flavoured olive oil
a few grinds of black pepper
20 basil leaves, roughly chopped

- Simply place all the ingredients, except the basil, in a blender and blitz for 12–15 seconds, or until smooth. Scrape into a bowl, stir the basil through and season to taste.
- Alternatively, you could blend the basil along with the rest of the ingredients to create a light green mayo.
- For the best flavour, make the mayo near serving time; it will keep in the fridge for a day or two.

Tips

If you don't have any sugar cane syrup, simply dissolve 1 teaspoon caster sugar in the lemon juice.

For a spicy mayo that pairs well with homemade avocado and vegetable sushi rolls, add a teaspoon or two of wasabi.

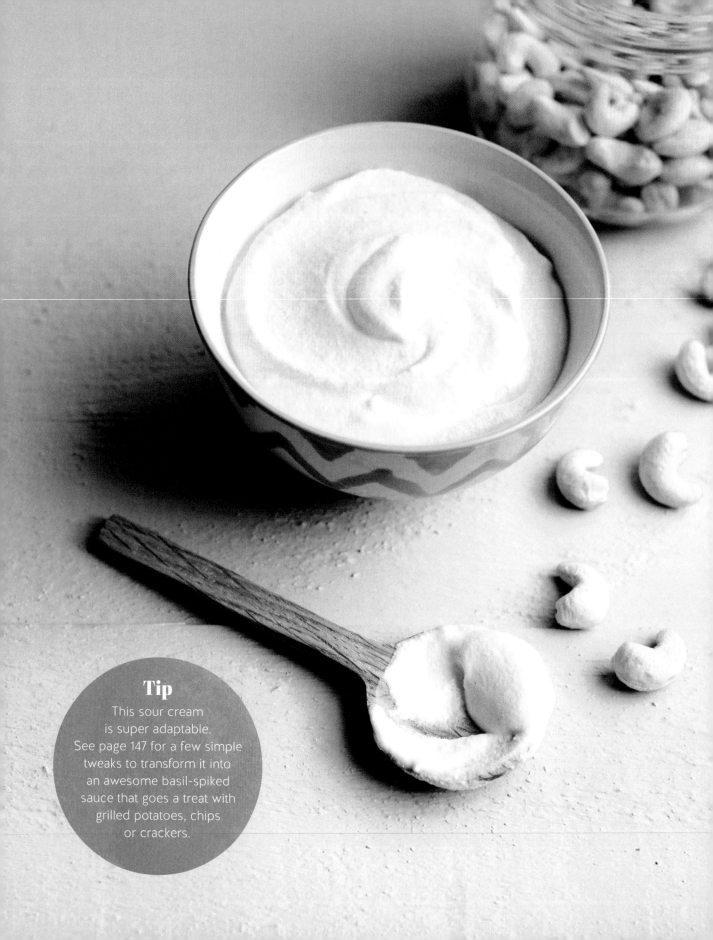

Tip

This sour cream is super adaptable. See page 147 for a few simple tweaks to transform it into an awesome basil-spiked sauce that goes a treat with grilled potatoes, chips or crackers.

Cashew Sour Cream

MAKES ABOUT 1-1½ CUPS

Silkily cool, rich and refreshing with a citrus tang, this cashew sour cream is perfect for dolloping on burritos, Smoky Southern black beans (page 222), Hungarian goulash (page 173) or Spicy bean nachos (page 172).

2 cups raw cashews
juice of 2 lemons
2 teaspoons apple cider vinegar
½ teaspoon salt
1-2 teaspoons nutritional yeast
   (optional, but recommended)

- Soak the cashews in water overnight. If you're short on time, place the cashews in a heatproof bowl, pour in enough boiling water to just cover them, then leave to soak for 1 hour, or a bit longer if you can – the end result won't be as silky smooth, but will still be creamier than using unsoaked cashews.

- Drain the cashews and place in a blender. Add ¾-1 cup water and the remaining ingredients, then blitz until the mixture is smooth and creamy.

- Check the seasoning, before scraping into a bowl, covering and chilling until required. The sour cream should keep for at least 5 days in the fridge.

Creamy Homestyle Tzatziki

MAKES ABOUT 2½ CUPS

One of the world's favourite dips, revamped to be 100% calf-friendly! Rich, cool and creamy, this dairy-free tzatziki is the perfect accompaniment to salads and falafel wraps, makes a great sandwich spread, and is delicious as part of an appetiser platter with some biscuits, raw vegies and crackers.

1½ cups plain, unsweetened
   coconut yoghurt
1 Lebanese cucumber, grated,
   then squeezed dry (see tip)
2-3 tablespoons chopped parsley
2-3 tablespoons chopped mint
2-3 tablespoons chopped dill
1-2 garlic cloves, crushed
zest and juice of 1 lemon

- Simply combine all the ingredients in a bowl and mix well. Season with salt and pepper to taste, going easy to begin with, remembering that lemon juice can make foods taste saltier than they are.

- Cover and refrigerate for at least 15 minutes, to allow the flavours to infuse.

- Give the tzatziki another good stir, check the seasoning, then spoon into a serving bowl and serve.

Tip
You can save the cucumber juice and add it to a Passion for greens smoothie (page 81).

Rich Mushroom Gravy

SERVES 4 GENEROUSLY (AND GRAVY SHOULD ALWAYS BE GENEROUS!)

Porcini mushrooms are the very essence of autumn: earthy, woodsy, with a strong savoury flavour that marries perfectly with thyme and marsala to create a rich gravy that can be poured over roast vegetables, creamy polenta or mashed potato and vegie sausages.

4 cups 'chicken-style' or 'beef-style' vegetable stock

4–6 dried porcini mushrooms

¼ cup good-quality olive oil

1 onion, roughly chopped

2 celery stalks, roughly chopped

2 carrots, roughly chopped

1 garlic clove, unpeeled and crushed

2 thyme sprigs

2 bay leaves (fresh, if possible)

1 tablespoon brown sugar

2 tablespoons plain flour

1 tablespoon marsala wine (or a dry white or red wine)

½–1 teaspoon vegetable yeast extract, such as Vegemite

1½ tablespoons soy sauce or tamari

- Pour the stock into a large saucepan and crumble the dried porcini mushrooms into it. Bring the mixture to the boil, then remove from the heat. Allow the mushrooms to infuse for at least 20 minutes (overnight is also fine – just bring back to room temperature before adding to the gravy).

- In a large, heavy-based saucepan, warm the olive oil over medium–high heat. Add the onion, celery, carrots, garlic, thyme and bay leaves. Sauté for 10–15 minutes, stirring occasionally, until the onion is starting to turn a caramelised gold. Add the sugar, stirring well until dissolved.

- Sprinkle the flour into the saucepan and stir constantly for 1 minute to allow the flour to cook off a little. Deglaze the pan with the marsala, then stir in the yeast extract and soy sauce.

- Strain the porcini vegetable stock, reserving the liquid, and discard the mushrooms. Slowly add the stock to the pan in a steady stream, and stir or whisk as though your life depends upon it – no one likes lumpy gravy, after all! Don't pour in the last few spoonfuls of stock if there's some mushroom grit in the bottom.

- Stirring constantly, bring the gravy back to the boil, then lower the heat to a gentle simmer and allow to reduce to the desired consistency. This could take up to 15 minutes – but good things usually do take time.

- Strain into another large saucepan and reheat if necessary. Taste for seasoning before pouring into a gravy boat and carrying your creation, steaming, to the table.

Variations

- This gravy can be easily transformed into a rich wine gravy: simply replace 1 cup of the vegetable stock with 1 cup dry white wine or red wine.

- For a hearty mushroom gravy that pairs deliciously with polenta or mashed potatoes, stir in, just before serving, some sliced mushrooms that have been sautéed with chopped garlic.

- You can also use dried shiitake mushrooms in place of the porcini mushrooms, but the flavour will be somewhat less intense.

Creamy Ranch Dressing

MAKES ABOUT 1¼ CUPS

This herby, uber-creamy dressing goes a treat with the Cauliflower buffalo 'wings' on page 100. And just about anything, really!

1 cup egg-free mayonnaise
1½ tablespoons dairy-free milk
2 teaspoons apple cider vinegar
1 teaspoon onion powder
¼ teaspoon sea salt
¼ teaspoon ground pepper
1 tablespoon finely chopped dill
1 tablespoon finely chopped parsley
1 tablespoon finely chopped chives

- In a bowl, whisk all the ingredients together until smooth. That's it!
- The dressing will keep in an airtight jar in the fridge for a few days.

Recipe contributed by hot for food

Tangy Butter Bean and Basil Dip

SERVES 6 AS AN APPETISER

Beautifully fresh-flavoured, this quick and easy dip can be served with crackers or corn chips, or even used to liven up toasted sandwiches. Try it inside burritos or on top of nachos – this delightful dip will make any Mexican dish sing! Spice it up by garnishing with fresh chopped chilli, or add extra lemon juice for extra tang.

1 tablespoon olive oil
1 garlic clove, crushed
400 g tin butterbeans, rinsed
   and drained
1 lemon
a pinch of chilli powder
a pinch of rock salt
2 tablespoons nutritional yeast
¼ cup finely chopped basil
1 avocado, mashed
balsamic vinegar, for drizzling

- Heat the oil in a frying pan over medium heat. Add the garlic and sauté for about 30 seconds, or until fragrant. Add the butterbeans and cook for 2 minutes, stirring occasionally.
- Grate the zest of the lemon and set aside. Juice the lemon and add half the juice to the pan, stirring quickly.
- Remove from the heat, then add the remaining lemon juice, along with the lemon zest, chilli powder, salt, nutritional yeast and basil.
- Mash the ingredients together using a potato masher, then leave to cool for a few minutes. Stir in the mashed avocado until mixed well, but still chunky. Alternatively, this dip can be blended to achieve a smoother, creamy consistency.
- Transfer to a serving bowl, drizzle with balsamic vinegar and serve.

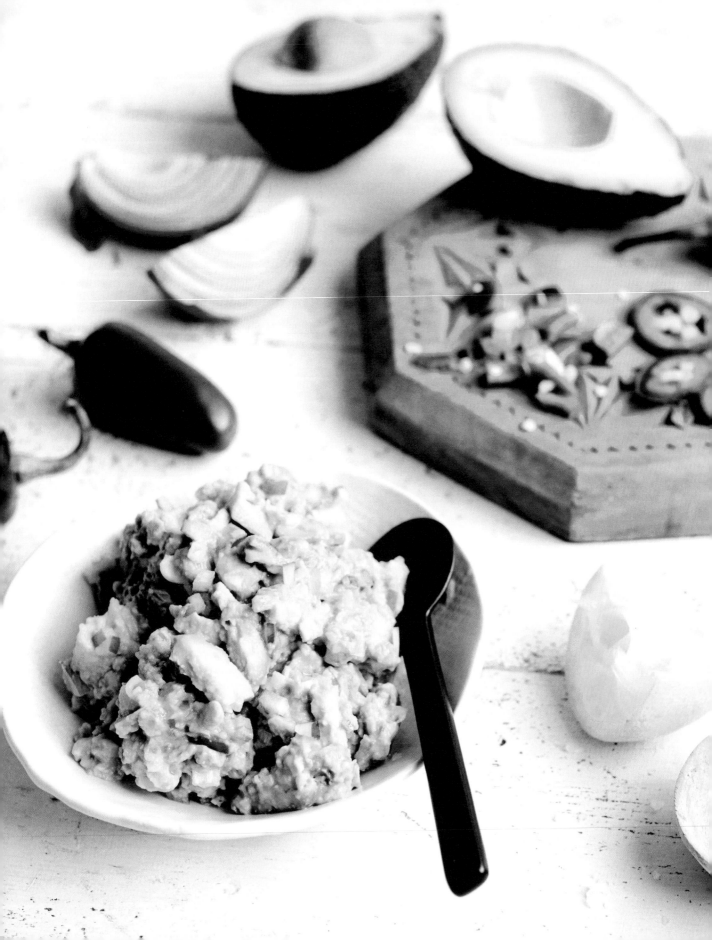

Guacamole

MAKES 2 CUPS

The zing in this classic guacamole comes straight from a jar of jalapeño chillies. Adding a little of the jalapeño pickling juice gives this guacamole a rich, authentic Mexican flavour, but you can use lime or lemon juice instead if you prefer. You can also add a finely chopped tomato and/or some finely chopped fresh coriander at the end.

2 large ripe avocados
1 tablespoon olive oil
1 garlic clove, crushed
½ teaspoon salt
1 tablespoon jalapeño pickling juice
　(from a jar of jalapeño chillies)
¼ large red onion, very finely chopped
3–5 pickled jalapeño chillies, finely
　chopped, to garnish (optional)

- Cut the avocados in half, remove the stones and scoop the flesh into a bowl. Add all the remaining ingredients, except the chopped jalapeños, and mash together, leaving some bits of avocado chunky if you like some texture in your guacamole.

- Alternatively, scoop the avocado into a food processor and add the olive oil, garlic, salt and jalapeño pickling juice. Pulse if you like your guacamole chunky, or blend if you like it smooth, adding the onion towards the end and pulsing just enough to mix it in.

- Garnish with the jalapeño chillies, if desired. Serve immediately.

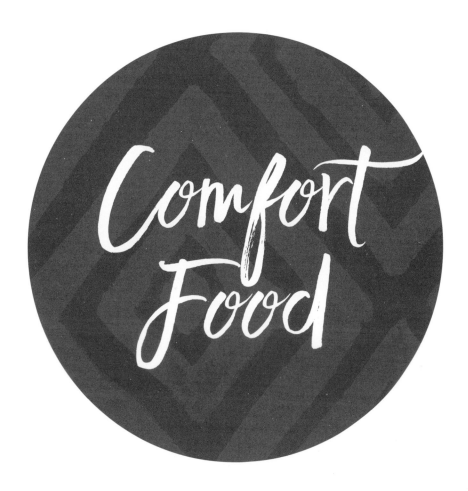

Comfort Food

Celebrate plant-based cuisine while still enjoying all the familiar meals
you grew up with. From pizza and spaghetti to lasagna and
even 'fish' and chips, we've taken some old favourites and given
them a tasty animal-friendly twist!

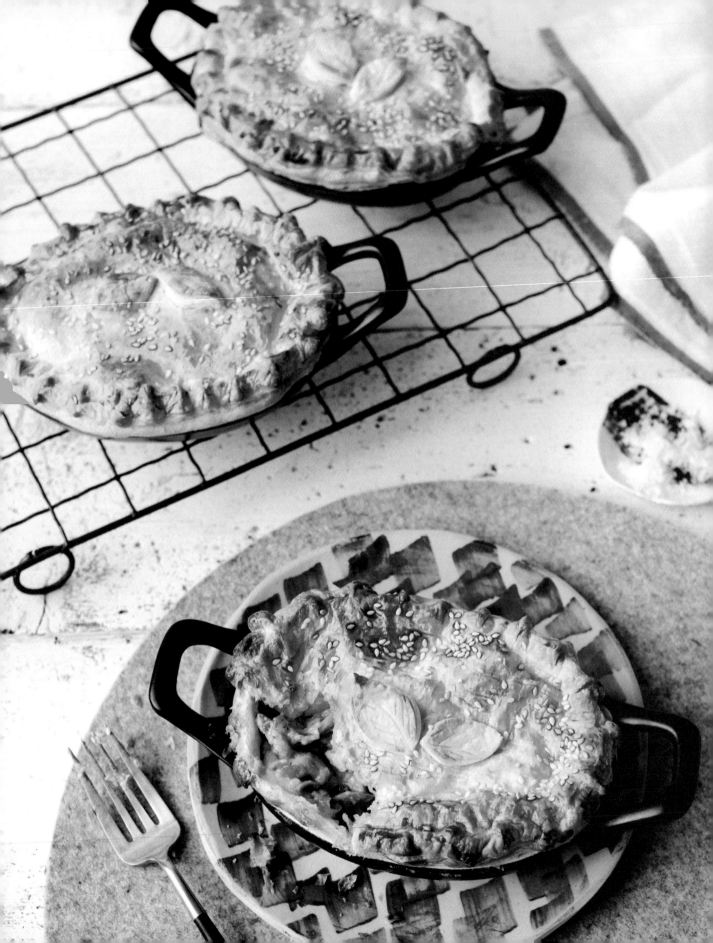

Mushroom and Leek Pie

SERVES 6

It's a cold winter's night and you're after a warm, hearty dinner – so what do you cook? A pie! With soft leek and mushrooms coated in a creamy sauce, all wrapped up in fluffy, crisp pastry, this pie is sure to satisfy. Serve with baked potatoes for carb-heaven, and some simple steamed greens on the side. Feel free to slather with your favourite sauce, gravy or relish before digging in.

1–2 tablespoons olive oil

6 garlic cloves, diced

1 leek, pale section only, sliced

700 g button mushrooms, wiped clean and sliced

4–5 spring onions, sliced

1 vegetable stock cube

1 teaspoon cracked black pepper

a large pinch of salt

5 sheets of frozen dairy-free puff pastry

WHITE SAUCE

4 tablespoons dairy-free margarine

4 tablespoons plain flour

2 cups soy milk

• Preheat the oven to 220°C conventional, or 200°C fan-forced.

• Heat the olive oil in a large frying pan over medium heat and sauté the garlic for 30 seconds, until aromatic. Add the leek, mushrooms and spring onions.

• Crumble the stock cube over the vegies, then stir frequently over medium heat for 5 minutes or so, until the liquid has reduced. Mix in the pepper and salt to taste. Set aside.

• To make the white sauce, melt the margarine in a large saucepan over medium heat. Add the flour and stir for about a minute, ensuring you press out any lumps of flour and thoroughly blend the mixture. Gradually add the soy milk, mixing in one splash at a time until you have a thick sauce. Once a thick gravy consistency is reached, add the mushroom and leek mixture and stir to combine. Remove from the heat and set aside.

• About 10 minutes before you plan to use them, take the puff pastry sheets out of the freezer and separate them. Once they have thawed, but while they are still cold, use them to line the base and sides of a large rectangular baking dish, measuring about 40 cm x 30 cm, and about 3 cm deep, leaving enough pastry to cover the top of the pie; you will probably need to cut the pastry to fit the dish. Transfer to the oven and bake for about 5–10 minutes, until the pastry is light golden brown.

• Remove the baking dish from the oven. Add the mushroom mixture, then lay a final sheet of puff pastry over the top. Return to the oven and bake for a further 15–25 minutes, until the pastry is puffed, cooked through and golden brown.

• Remove from the oven and allow to stand for 5 minutes before serving.

Tip

Instead of baking the pie in one big dish, you could use six small baking dishes or ramekins. You won't need to cook the individual pies as long. Refer to the pastry packet instructions for general cooking times.

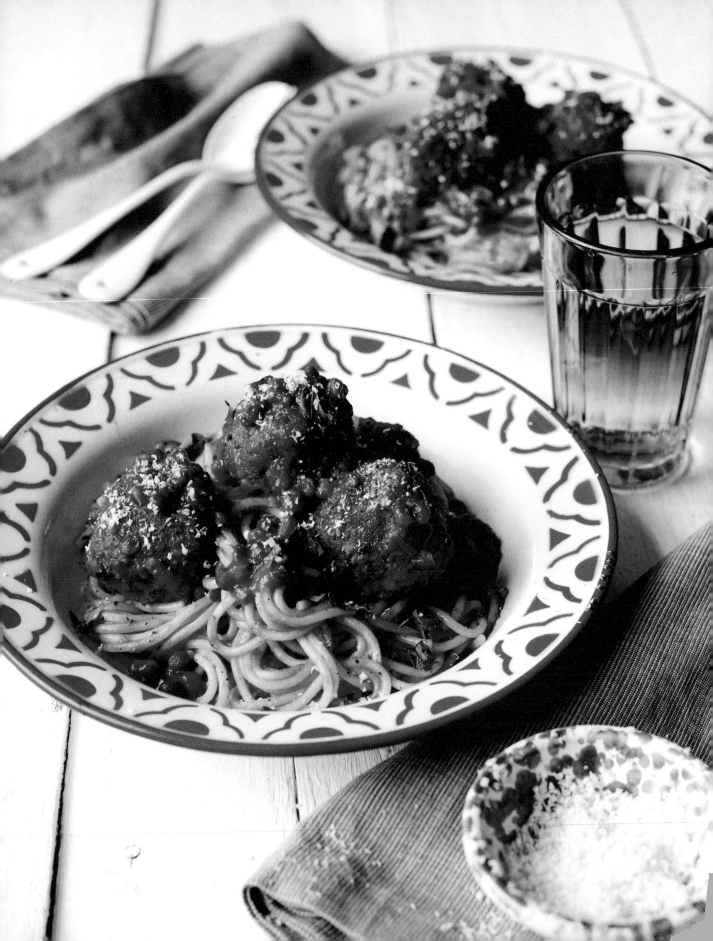

Bolognaise with No-meat Balls

SERVES 4

There's only one thing more comforting than a steaming bowl of pasta and that's knowing that it's cruelty-free. This delicious meat-free version of everyone's favourite will have the whole family asking for seconds.

vegetable oil, for pan-frying
500 g spaghetti, or your favourite pasta
Cashew parmesan (page 187),
    or dairy-free cheese, to serve

LENTIL BOLOGNAISE

1 tablespoon olive oil
1 large brown onion, diced
2 garlic cloves, crushed
1 teaspoon salt
2 teaspoons dried thyme
1 teaspoon chilli flakes
1 teaspoon dried basil
400 g tin brown lentils, drained
1 carrot, grated
400 g tin diced tomatoes
400 g tin tomato soup

NO-MEAT BALLS

1 tablespoon ground flaxseeds
3 tablespoons warm water
300 g block of tempeh
2 French shallots, chopped
2 garlic cloves, peeled
2 tablespoons vegan
    Worcestershire sauce
2 tablespoons Cashew parmesan
    (page 187) or nutritional yeast
2 tablespoons chopped parsley
1 tablespoon dried oregano
1 teaspoon dried basil
1 teaspoon salt
⅓ cup breadcrumbs, plus extra
    for coating the balls

• To make the bolognaise, heat the olive oil in a large saucepan over medium heat, add the onion and cook for 2 minutes, or until soft and translucent. Stir in the garlic, salt, thyme, chilli and basil and cook for 1 minute, or until fragrant. Add the lentils and carrot and cook for a further 2 minutes, or until the carrot is soft and heated through.

• Stir in the tomatoes and tomato soup, and add up to 1 cup water to reach a saucy consistency. Bring to the boil, stirring continuously, then reduce the heat and leave to simmer for about 30 minutes, stirring regularly.

• Meanwhile, get started on the no-meat balls. In a small mug, mix together the flaxseeds and warm water. Leave to sit for about 10 minutes, or until the mixture turns into a gel.

• Break up the tempeh and place in a food processor. Add the shallots, garlic, Worcestershire sauce and cashew parmesan. Process until combined. Add the herbs, salt, flaxseed mixture and breadcrumbs and blend until well combined.

• Spread an extra ¼ cup breadcrumbs on a plate. Using a spoon, scoop up some of the tempeh mixture and roll it into a ball about the size of a golf ball. Roll the tempeh ball in the breadcrumbs so that it's completely covered, then set aside on a plate. Continue rolling and coating more balls, until all the tempeh mixture is used.

• Heat some vegetable oil in a large frying pan over medium–high heat. Working in batches if necessary, as you don't want to overcrowd the pan, cook the tempeh balls for about 10 minutes, gently shaking the pan now and then so they brown on all sides. (The balls are quite fragile, so shaking the pan to roll them around is easier than trying to turn them with a utensil.) When they are all browned, transfer the balls to a plate lined with paper towel; you can keep them warm in the oven, if you like.

• Meanwhile, cook the spaghetti according to the packet instructions. Drain, then toss the pasta through the bolognaise sauce.

• Divide among serving bowls, then top with the no-meat balls. Sprinkle with cashew parmesan or dairy-free cheese and serve.

No-Meat Balls recipe contributed by Rhea Parsons

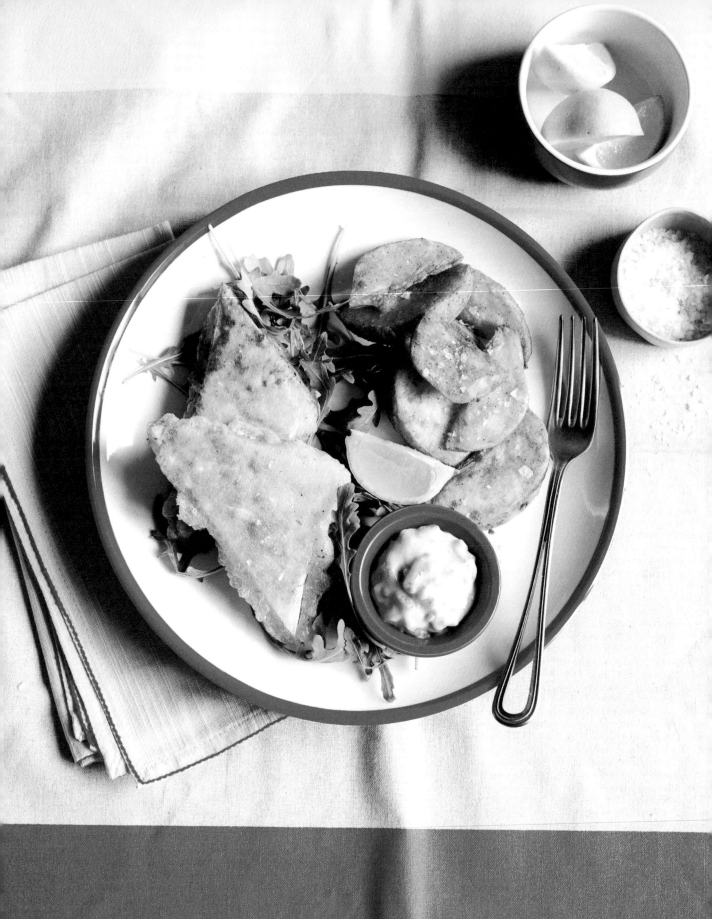

Beer-battered Tofish with Tartare Sauce

SERVES 2-3

Whether you're hungry, hangry or hungover, a big plate of these is the ultimate cure – delightful bite-sized triangles of marinated tofu, salty with a hint of the sea, encased in a crunchy, airy beer batter. The recipe is simple and the results are exactly what you've been craving. We recommend serving with Spicy potato wedges (page 112), and perhaps a salad to add some greenery.

250 g firm tofu
2 teaspoons kelp powder (available
   from health food stores)
2 teaspoons garlic powder
½ teaspoon sweet paprika
2 teaspoons salt
1–2 tablespoons olive oil
lemon wedges, to serve
rice bran oil or grapeseed oil,
   for shallow-frying

TARTARE SAUCE

3–4 tablespoons egg-free mayonnaise
4–5 gherkins or dill pickles,
   finely diced
juice of ½ lemon

BEER BATTER

1½ cups plain flour
375 ml bottle of light beer,
   such as a pilsener

- Slice the tofu in half widthways, and in half again lengthways. Then slice the four pieces into two triangles by cutting each piece diagonally. You should end up with 8 tofu triangles, but there are no hard and fast rules here – cut out stars if you like!

- Make a marinade by combining the kelp powder, garlic powder, paprika, salt and olive oil in a bowl. Add the tofu pieces and gently mix to coat, then cover and marinate in the fridge for at least 2 hours, or preferably overnight.

- Meanwhile, combine all the tartare sauce ingredients in an airtight container and store in the fridge until you're ready to serve.

- Just before serving, prepare the batter. Simply put the flour in a bowl, pour the beer over and whisk gently until just combined.

- Heat a heavy-based frying pan or wok over medium–high heat. Add enough rice bran oil to cover the base. Working in batches, to avoid overcrowding the pan or wok, dip the tofu pieces in the batter, covering them generously, then cook for about 5 minutes on each side, until light brown and crispy, being careful when flipping them over. Remove and drain on paper towel.

- Serve immediately, with lemon wedges and your tartare sauce.

Recipe contributed by Bed & Broccoli - Nikki Medwell

Spicy Bean Nachos

SERVES 2

It's the nachos you know and love – revamped as a calf-friendly, corn-chip comfort-food extravaganza! Spicy beans piled high atop a crunchy mountain of corn chips, peppered with sweet corn and melting dairy-free cheese, and it's hasta la vista, baby – except you'll soon be back for more.

1 tablespoon vegetable oil

1 brown onion, diced

1 tablespoon Taco seasoning mix (see recipe below)

400 g tin four-bean mix, rinsed and drained

1 large ripe tomato, diced

230 g packet corn chips

100 g dairy-free cheese, grated (optional)

1 cup sweet corn kernels, rinsed and drained

Guacamole (page 163), to serve

small handful of coriander, roughly chopped

pickled jalapeño chilli slices, to serve (optional)

TACO SEASONING MIX

½ teaspoon onion powder

½ teaspoon garlic powder

½ teaspoon chilli flakes

1 teaspoon dried oregano

2 teaspoons sweet paprika

1 teaspoon ground cumin

a pinch of sea salt

a pinch of black pepper

- Combine all the taco seasoning mix ingredients in a small bowl and set aside.

- Heat the oil in a large saucepan and fry the onion over medium heat for 1–2 minutes, until softened and slightly translucent. Add the taco seasoning mix and stir for about 30 seconds, until all the aromas are released. Add the beans and stir to coat with the spice mix, then stir in the tomato and cook for 4–5 minutes, stirring frequently until slightly thickened.

- To serve, arrange the corn chips on a plate, then scatter with the cheese, if using. Top with the hot bean mix, sprinkle with the corn kernels and dollop on a generous spoonful of guacamole. Garnish with the coriander and serve with a small bowl of jalapeños on the side, for those who like to play it hot.

Tips

If you're short on spices, you can use a packet of taco mix from the supermarket – we won't tell …

For an easy 'chilli sin carne', swap out the corn chips for a whole baked potato or sweet potato.

Hungarian Goulash

SERVES 4

Few dishes showcase paprika better than a traditional Hungarian goulash, and here the combination of sweet and spicy provides the perfect balance of flavours. The mushrooms, potatoes and carrots make this a hearty dish, but you can add any combination of vegetables, or even beans – butterbeans are especially delicious! The small homemade noodles ('nokedli') are the traditional accompaniment to a goulash, and so easy to make – but you can serve with noodles or rice if you prefer.

2 tablespoons grapeseed oil

1 large brown onion, chopped

½ red capsicum, seeded and chopped

1 kg mixed mushrooms (portobello and button mushrooms are good!), sliced or quartered depending on size

3 garlic cloves, peeled

1 teaspoon caraway seeds

3 tablespoons sweet Hungarian paprika

1 teaspoon hot Hungarian paprika (optional)

2 large potatoes, peeled and chopped into 3 cm chunks

1 large carrot, chopped into 3 cm chunks

400 g tin whole peeled tomatoes

2–3 cups vegetable stock

1 bay leaf

1 tablespoon cornflour (optional)

NOKEDLI

2 tablespoons sunflower oil, plus extra for drizzling

1 heaped tablespoon semolina

1 cup plain flour

a pinch of vegetable stock powder

To make the goulash, heat the grapeseed oil in a large saucepan, then fry the onion and capsicum over medium heat, stirring occasionally, for about 5 minutes, until soft. Add the mushrooms and season to taste with salt and pepper. Cook for about 8 minutes, until soft and browned, stirring now and then. Don't drain the water that comes out of the mushrooms, as it will add to the final flavour.

Crush the garlic cloves. You can also crush the caraway seeds using a mortar and pestle, or leave them whole – or crush some to release their flavour, and leave the rest whole for texture. Mix the crushed garlic and caraway seeds to make a paste. Stir in a pinch of salt, then add the garlicky caraway paste to the saucepan with the sweet and hot paprika. Stir for a few minutes, allowing the paprika to release all its flavour.

Add the potatoes, carrot, tomatoes, vegetable stock and bay leaf. Stir until combined, then bring to the boil.

Cover, reduce the heat to low and simmer for 30 minutes, or until the potatoes are cooked through. At this point, you can choose to add the cornflour, blended to a smooth paste with some of the pan juices, to thicken the sauce, or leave as is. Keep warm.

While the goulash is simmering, bring a medium to large saucepan of salted water to the boil.

Combine the noodle ingredients in a mixing bowl. Using a wooden spoon, gradually mix in ½ cup cold water until the mixture becomes soft and a little gluey, and the consistency of pancake batter.

Hold the bowl over the boiling water and drip the mixture into the pot, using a knife to separate the drips; they will form into noodles instantly. The noodle drips can be big or small, and they'll all be different in shape, but try to keep them roughly the same size so they cook evenly. The noodles are cooked when they float to the top. Lift them out using a slotted spoon and place into a bowl. Stir in a little extra oil so they don't stick together.

Divide the warm noodles among serving bowls, top with generous spoonfuls of the goulash and serve.

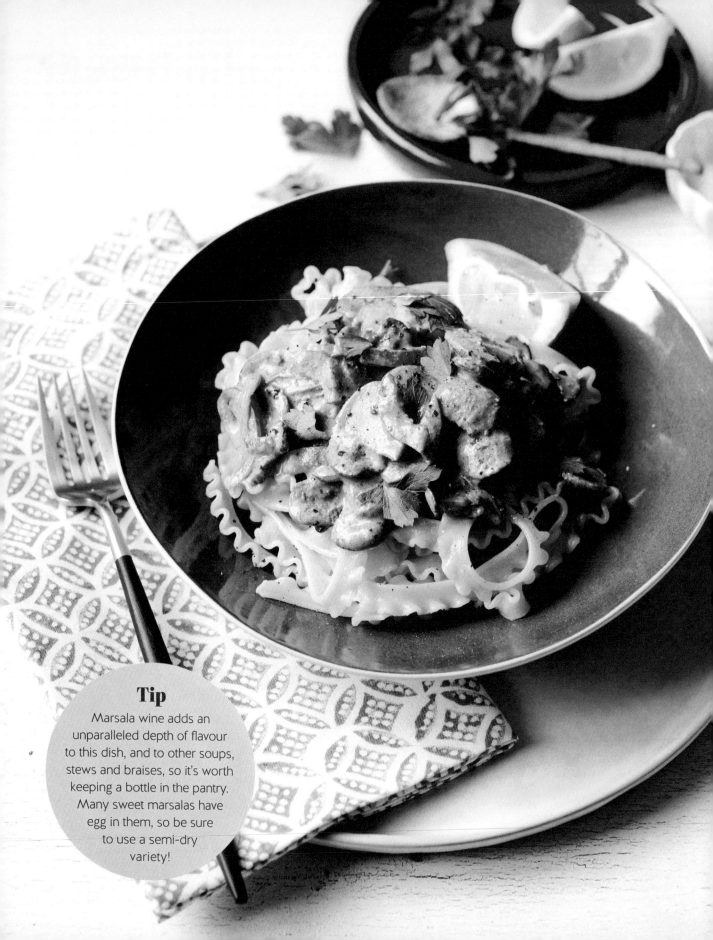

Tip

Marsala wine adds an unparalleled depth of flavour to this dish, and to other soups, stews and braises, so it's worth keeping a bottle in the pantry. Many sweet marsalas have egg in them, so be sure to use a semi-dry variety!

Rich Mushroom Stroganoff

SERVES 4

A scattering of fresh herbs enlivens this hearty dish, richly flavoured with smoked paprika. Creamy and voluptuous, it is delicious served with pasta, rice or simply hot crusty bread. Double or even triple the ingredients and enjoy with friends.

3 tablespoons olive oil

500 g button mushrooms, thickly sliced

2 large brown onions, halved and thinly sliced

1 small green capsicum, thinly sliced (optional)

½ teaspoon dried thyme

½ teaspoon dried sage

½ teaspoon dried dill

2–4 tablespoons smoked paprika, to taste

½ teaspoon chilli flakes (optional)

3 garlic cloves, crushed

2 tablespoons semi-dry marsala wine (see tip)

1 tablespoon tomato paste, dissolved in 1 cup water

2 tablespoons vegan Worcestershire sauce

chopped parsley or dill, to garnish

lemon wedges, to serve

CASHEW CREAM

¾ cup raw cashews, soaked in 1 cup boiling water for at least 15 minutes

1 teaspoon vegetable stock powder

½–¾ cup full-cream soy milk

2 teaspoons apple cider vinegar or red wine vinegar (optional)

Warm 2 tablespoons of the olive oil in a large, deep frying pan over medium heat. Add the mushrooms and cook, stirring occasionally, for about 5–7 minutes, until most of the mushrooms have some brown edges. (If you put all the mushrooms in at once, they may steam rather than fry, releasing their flavoursome juices; just pour the juices into a bowl to add back in later, and keep on frying.) Transfer the cooked mushrooms to a plate and set aside.

Warm the remaining tablespoon of oil in the frying pan and sauté the onions for about 5 minutes, until translucent.

Add the capsicum, if using, then sprinkle with the dried herbs and give it a quick stir before adding the paprika. Add the chilli flakes now, if using. Fry for 30 seconds, or until fragrant, then add the garlic and stir for a further 30 seconds.

Stir the mushrooms back in, then deglaze the pan with the marsala, stirring well. Pour in the tomato paste mixture, along with any reserved mushroom juices. Add the Worcestershire sauce and plenty of black pepper, give everything a good stir to combine well, then leave to simmer for 10–15 minutes, to allow all the flavours to infuse.

While the stroganoff is simmering, prepare the cashew cream. Place the cashews and their soaking liquid in a blender, add the remaining cashew cream ingredients and blitz on high speed until smooth and creamy.

When you're ready to serve, stir the cashew cream through the stroganoff. Bring the mixture to a simmer to heat through.

Sprinkle with the parsley or dill and serve immediately, with your choice of accompaniment, and lemon wedges on the side.

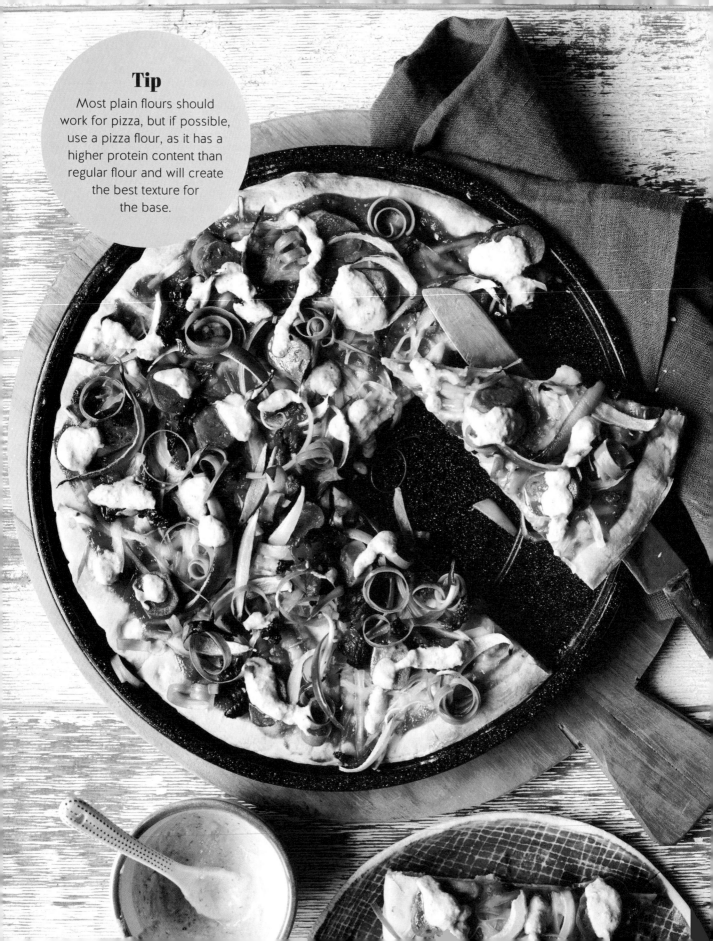

Tip

Most plain flours should work for pizza, but if possible, use a pizza flour, as it has a higher protein content than regular flour and will create the best texture for the base.

Meat-free-lovers' Barbecue Pizza

MAKES 2 MEDIUM PIZZAS

With infinite topping and flavour combinations, pizza is a great way to enjoy animal-friendly food. The mix of barbecue sauce and sundried tomatoes makes this pizza delightfully tangy; the addition of vegetarian sausage turns it into a meat-free-lovers' classic. Making your own dough is unbelievably simple, or you can buy a pizza base if you're short on time.

10 g dried yeast (less than roughly two 7 g sachets)

1 teaspoon sugar

3 cups pizza flour, approximately (see tip)

300 ml lukewarm water

2 tablespoons olive oil, plus a little extra for greasing

PIZZA TOPPING

4 tablespoons tomato paste

½ cup barbecue sauce

½ cup grated dairy-free cheese, such as Biocheese (because it melts well)

4 vegan hot dogs, sliced at an angle into 1 cm pieces

1 red onion, thinly sliced

½ cup finely chopped sundried tomatoes

chopped or sliced and curled spring onions, to garnish (optional)

Herbed sour cream (page 147), to drizzle (optional)

Combine the yeast, sugar and 1 heaped tablespoon of the flour in a small mixing bowl. Stir in the warm water, then cover and leave in a warm place for 15 minutes, until the mixture is foamy.

Meanwhile, heat the oven to its highest setting: 250°C conventional, or 230°C fan-forced if possible, or at least 220°C conventional, 200°C fan-forced. Place two pizza trays in the oven to heat up.

Put 2½ cups of the flour in a large mixing bowl with a pinch of salt. Mix together, making a well in the centre. Slowly add the warm yeast mixture, along with the olive oil. Mix with your hand until a smooth dough forms, adding a little more flour if needed to make the dough less sticky.

Grease a large mixing bowl with olive oil. Add the dough and cover with a clean damp tea towel. Set aside in a warm place to rise for 30 minutes, or up to 60 minutes. The dough should at least double in size.

Divide the dough into two balls, trying not to knock out too much air. Carefully stretch and flatten each dough ball out to a round pizza shape and place on your hot pizza trays.

Transfer the pizza bases to the hot oven and bake without any toppings for 5–7 minutes, depending on how hot your oven is. You want the outside crust to just start to firm. Carefully remove from the oven – the pizza bases will be very hot!

Spread each base with the tomato paste, then half the barbecue sauce. Layer the grated cheese, hot dog slices, onion and sundried tomato on each base, then drizzle with the remaining barbecue sauce. (Dairy-free cheese tends to cook a little differently, so always put it as the bottom layer in a pizza for maximum meltiness.)

Bake for a further 10–15 minutes, or until the crust is golden brown – keep an eye on the pizzas to ensure they don't burn.

Remove from the oven. Scatter with spring onions and drizzle with Herbed sour cream if desired. Cut, serve and enjoy.

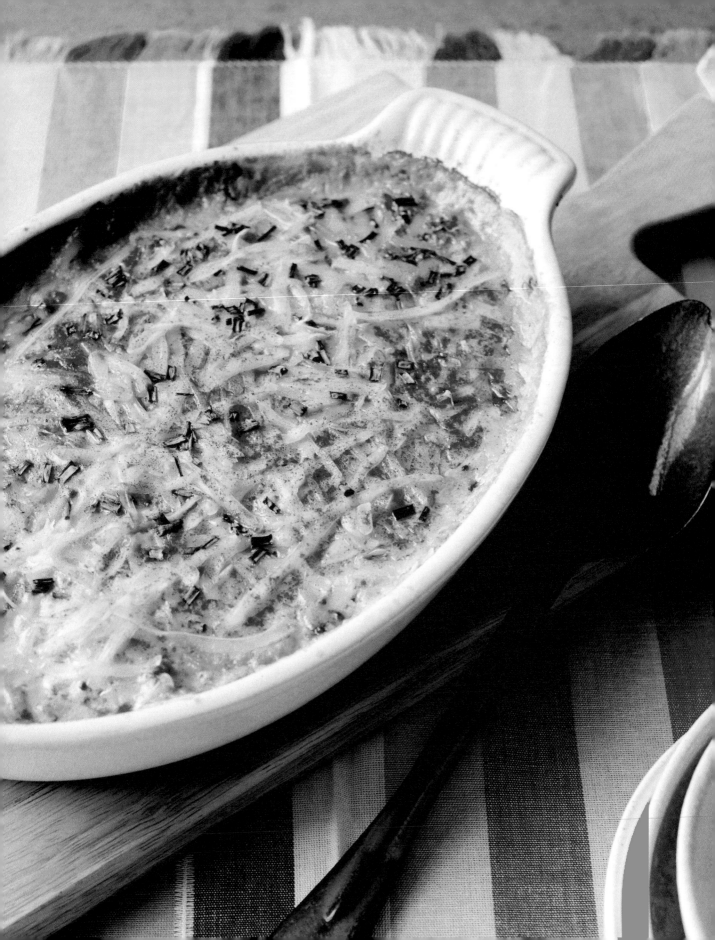

Creamy Potato Bake

SERVES 4-6

This incredibly easy, no-fuss potato bake is a real comforter in winter, but is also delicious served cold at a summer barbecue. Delightfully creamy, it's guaranteed to satisfy all your potato cravings.

2 tablespoons olive oil
4 large potatoes
300 g silken tofu
1½ cups unsweetened soy milk
2 garlic cloves, crushed
1 tablespoon soy sauce
1 teaspoon mustard powder
½ cup nutritional yeast
½ x 40 g packet dairy-free French
   onion soup mix (about 4 teaspoons)
   (see tip)
100 g dairy-free cheese, grated
½ teaspoon sweet paprika
1 tablespoon chopped chives

- Preheat the oven to 200°C conventional, or 180°C fan-forced. Grease the base and side of a 1.5 litre baking dish or pie dish with 1 tablespoon of the olive oil.

- Peel the potatoes and cut into slices 5 mm thick. Place in a large saucepan and cover with cold water. Bring to the boil over high heat, then leave to boil for 5-7 minutes, or until the slices are fork tender, but not falling apart. Drain carefully into a colander and set aside.

- While the potatoes are boiling, make up a creamy sauce. Put the remaining olive oil in a food processor or blender, along with the tofu, soy milk, garlic, soy sauce, mustard powder and nutritional yeast. Season with salt and pepper and blend until smooth and creamy.

- Spread one layer of potato slices in the bottom of the baking dish. Pour a layer of sauce over, to just cover the potato slices. Sprinkle with about 1 teaspoon of the French onion soup mix, and one-quarter of the cheese. Continue this layering process until all the potato slices have been used, making sure you cover the final layer with the creamy sauce.

- Sprinkle with the paprika, then cover the dish with a lid or foil. To avoid cleaning-up hassles, place a baking tray under the baking dish, then pop the whole thing in the oven and bake for 40 minutes.

- Remove the lid or foil and bake for a further 15 minutes. The sauce will bubble and boil and appear runny when you remove the dish hot from the oven, but will thicken to a creamy consistency if left to cool for a few minutes before serving.

- Sprinkle with the chives, and enjoy warm or cold.

Tip
The remaining French onion soup mix will keep for a few weeks in an airtight container.

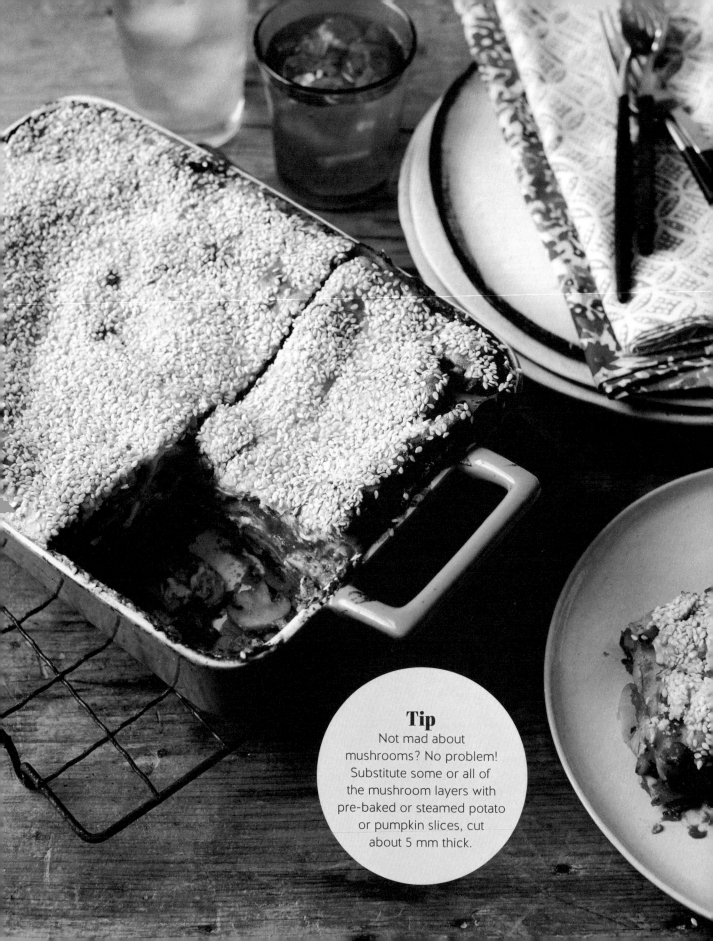

Tip
Not mad about mushrooms? No problem! Substitute some or all of the mushroom layers with pre-baked or steamed potato or pumpkin slices, cut about 5 mm thick.

Mushroom and Spinach Lasagne

SERVES 6-8

This saucy lasagne is much healthier than most, yet the recipe is as simple as its flavours are deliciously complex. It is perfect for a large family dinner, or an impressive dinner party dish, as you can even make the tomato and béchamel sauces the day before – in fact, it will taste even better if you do. Serve this layered creation with garlic-roasted potatoes for a maximum dose of comfort, and a crisp, green garden salad to round it all out.

375 g packet egg-free instant
    lasagne sheets
6 cups sliced mushrooms (see tip)
6 cups baby spinach leaves
¼ cup sesame seeds

HERBED TOMATO SAUCE

2 tablespoons olive oil, plus extra
    for greasing
1 large onion, chopped
2 large garlic cloves, crushed
700–750 g jar tomato passata
400 g tin chopped tomatoes
1 tablespoon dried oregano
1 tablespoon dried basil
1 teaspoon salt
½ cup vegetable stock or water,
    approximately
400 g tin cooked lentils, drained
    and rinsed

BÉCHAMEL SAUCE

500 g silken tofu, drained
2 cups raw cashews
½ cup lemon juice
⅓ cup olive oil
2 garlic cloves, peeled
2 teaspoons salt

- Preheat the oven to 200°C conventional, or 180°C fan-forced. Grease a lasagne baking dish with olive oil.

- To make the tomato sauce, heat the olive oil in a large saucepan over medium heat and fry the onion for 5 minutes, or until translucent. Add the garlic and fry for a further 1 minute, then add the remaining sauce ingredients, stirring well. Season with pepper, bring to a simmer and leave to bubble away for 10 minutes. If the sauce is very thick, stir in an extra ¼–½ cup stock or water.

- Meanwhile, put all the béchamel sauce ingredients in a blender. Simply blitz on high speed until smooth and creamy.

- To assemble the lasagne, ladle about one-quarter of the tomato sauce into the bottom of the dish. Begin layering with the mushrooms, then the spinach, béchamel and pasta sheets. Continue layering until all the ingredients are used up – making sure you finish with a layer of béchamel. Sprinkle the top of the lasagne with the sesame seeds.

- Bake, uncovered, for 40 minutes, or until a knife will slide easily through the pasta layers.

- Remove from the oven and leave to stand for 10 minutes before serving.

- This lasagne can be made the day before; sitting overnight helps the flavours combine to give an even tastier dish. This also helps with serving, giving all the layers time to set. Simply cut into portions, cover the individual serves and reheat in the oven for 10–15 minutes.

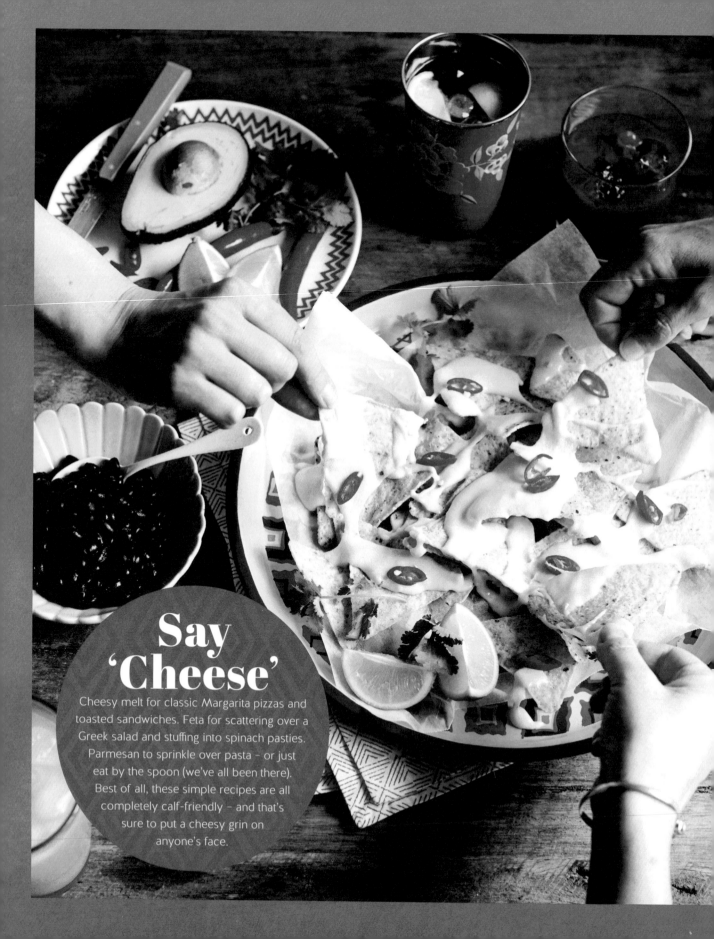

Say 'Cheese'

Cheesy melt for classic Margarita pizzas and toasted sandwiches. Feta for scattering over a Greek salad and stuffing into spinach pasties. Parmesan to sprinkle over pasta – or just eat by the spoon (we've all been there). Best of all, these simple recipes are all completely calf-friendly – and that's sure to put a cheesy grin on anyone's face.

Stretchy Gooey Cheesy Melt

MAKES ABOUT 1 CUP

This soft, versatile cheese can be used in so many ways – on top of nachos, dolloped onto pizza before baking, in a toasted cheese sandwich, or however your cheese-loving heart desires. It will keep in the fridge for several days.

½ cup raw cashews
3½ tablespoons tapioca starch
 (see tip)
1 tablespoon nutritional yeast
1 teaspoon apple cider vinegar
½ teaspoon salt
¼ teaspoon garlic powder

- If you don't have a high-powered blender, you will first need to boil or soak the cashews to soften them. To soak the cashews, cover them with cold water and soak for 4 hours, or overnight. To boil the cashews, place them in a saucepan, cover with cold water, bring to the boil and cook for 10–15 minutes, or until they are tender and can be easily broken between your fingers. Drain the cashews and add them to a blender, along with 1 cup water.

- Add all the remaining ingredients to the blender and blitz until completely smooth. The mixture will be very watery. (If you didn't use a high-powered blender, you may want to pour the liquid through a fine-mesh strainer or cheesecloth before cooking it, to remove any cashew bits that didn't grind up; this will ensure a smooth cheese texture.)

- Pour the mixture into a small saucepan and place over medium-high heat. Stir continuously as the mixture cooks. As you stir it will start forming clumps – and then all of a sudden it will become a cheesy, gooey mass of yumminess. This takes about 5 minutes.

- Continue cooking and stirring for a further 2 minutes, to make sure it has firmed up completely.

- Use straight away, in any recipe where you'd like a melty cheese.

- Alternatively, store it in an airtight container in the fridge. To bring the cold mozzarella back to a dipping consistency, gently reheat over medium heat, stirring constantly so it doesn't burn. Once it is hot and bubbling, it might have thickened up too much, but you can thin it out by adding a tablespoon of water at a time, stirring it in until the desired consistency is reached.

Tip
Also known as tapioca flour, tapioca starch is essential for this recipe. It is what gives the cheese its gooey and stretchy texture.

Recipe contributed by Sam Turnbull

Cheesy Corn Brunch Muffins

MAKES 12 MUFFINS

These savoury muffins are easy to whip up, and are a tasty option if you don't have a sweet tooth in the morning. Nutritional yeast may sound a little strange, but it simply adds a cheesy bite, as well as loads of goodness. This basic mix is simple to tweak to your tastes – see the variations at the end of the recipe for a few ideas.

a large handful of baby spinach leaves
½ cup soy milk
1 tablespoon apple cider vinegar
4 tablespoons olive oil
¾ cup creamed corn
½ cup dry instant polenta
1 cup plain flour
2 teaspoons baking powder
1 teaspoon sweet or smoked paprika
1–1½ teaspoons onion powder
1–1½ teaspoons garlic powder
½ teaspoon salt
a pinch of cayenne pepper or chilli flakes (optional)
2 teaspoons nutritional yeast (optional)
6 spring onions, chopped or a few tablespoons chopped chives
50 g grated dairy-free cheese (optional)

- Preheat the oven to 220°C conventional, or 200°C fan-forced. Line a 12-hole non-stick muffin tin with paper cases.

- Microwave or sauté the baby spinach with a teaspoon of water until just wilted; this will only take 20 seconds or so. Plunge into cold water to stop the cooking process and retain its lovely emerald green colour, then roughly chop and set aside.

- In a small bowl, mix together the soy milk and vinegar. Set aside to thicken for a few minutes, then mix in the olive oil and creamed corn.

- In a separate bowl, combine the polenta, flour, baking powder, paprika, onion powder, garlic powder, salt and a pinch of black pepper. Add the cayenne pepper and nutritional yeast, if using, and mix together well.

- Fold the chopped spinach and spring onions into the creamed corn mixture, along with the grated cheese, if using. Pour over the dry ingredients and stir together quickly and gently – just enough to combine. Overmixing will result in dense, tough muffins, so it's better to undermix than overmix; some dry patches are perfectly okay.

- Quickly spoon the mixture into the muffin cases. Bake for 15–20 minutes, or until the tops are golden.

- Best served warm, straight out of the oven.

Variations: To add a Mediterranean twist, fold through a handful of chopped sundried tomatoes, kalamata olives and a pinch of dried oregano with the wilted spinach – or simply top each muffin with half a fresh cherry tomato before baking. To spice things up, add 2 teaspoons wholegrain mustard to the soy milk and vinegar mixture.

Nacho Queso Dip

SERVES 4-6

Ideal for entertaining or a simple Sunday afternoon snack, this dip is based on a marriage made in heaven: creamy cashews and zesty salsa. Serve with corn chips, or vegetable sticks such as carrot, capsicum or celery.

1 cup chopped carrot

1 cup raw cashews

¼ cup nutritional yeast

2 tablespoons lemon juice

1 garlic clove, peeled

1½ teaspoons salt

½ teaspoon chilli powder, or to taste (optional)

450 g chunky salsa (if using a spicy one, don't add the chilli powder above)

½ cup grated dairy-free cheese or dairy-free sour cream (optional)

½ red onion, finely chopped

1 cup baby spinach leaves, firmly packed

- Preheat the oven to 200°C conventional, or 180°C fan-forced.
- Steam or microwave the carrots until soft. Leave to cool slightly, then place in a blender with the cashews, nutritional yeast, lemon juice, garlic, salt and chilli powder, if using. Add 1 cup water and blend on high until very smooth.
- Scrape the mixture into a large mixing bowl. Add the remaining ingredients and stir until well combined. Pour into a medium-sized baking dish and bake for 15 minutes. Cover with foil to stop the top burning, then bake for a further 5–10 minutes, until heated through.
- Remove from the oven, remove the foil and allow to cool slightly. Serve warm.
- Leftovers (if there are any!) will keep in the fridge for a few days. To serve, cover with foil and gently reheat in the oven.

Mac 'n' Cheese

SERVES 4

There are just five ingredients in this rich and creamy dairy-free version of an old favourite. But, as you'll quickly discover, less sometimes really is more. Serve with salad for a quick and easy mid-week meal.

1½ cups macaroni

1 tablespoon grapeseed oil

1 brown onion, finely diced

500 g tin condensed, dairy-free tomato soup

200 g dairy-free cheese, grated

- Preheat the oven to 180°C conventional, or 160°C fan-forced.
- Bring a saucepan of water to the boil. Add the macaroni and cook according to the packet instructions.
- Meanwhile, heat the grapeseed oil in a large, non-stick frying pan. Add the onion and fry over medium heat for about 5 minutes, until it turns a burnished golden brown. Add the tomato soup, then mix in most of the grated cheese, leaving some aside to sprinkle on top.
- When the macaroni is cooked, drain well and add to the pan. Mix well for 2–3 minutes, so the pasta has a chance to soak up all the flavours. Season with salt and pepper, to taste. Transfer the mixture to a baking dish, then sprinkle the reserved cheese over the top. Bake for 15–20 minutes, or until the macaroni is slightly crispy on top.

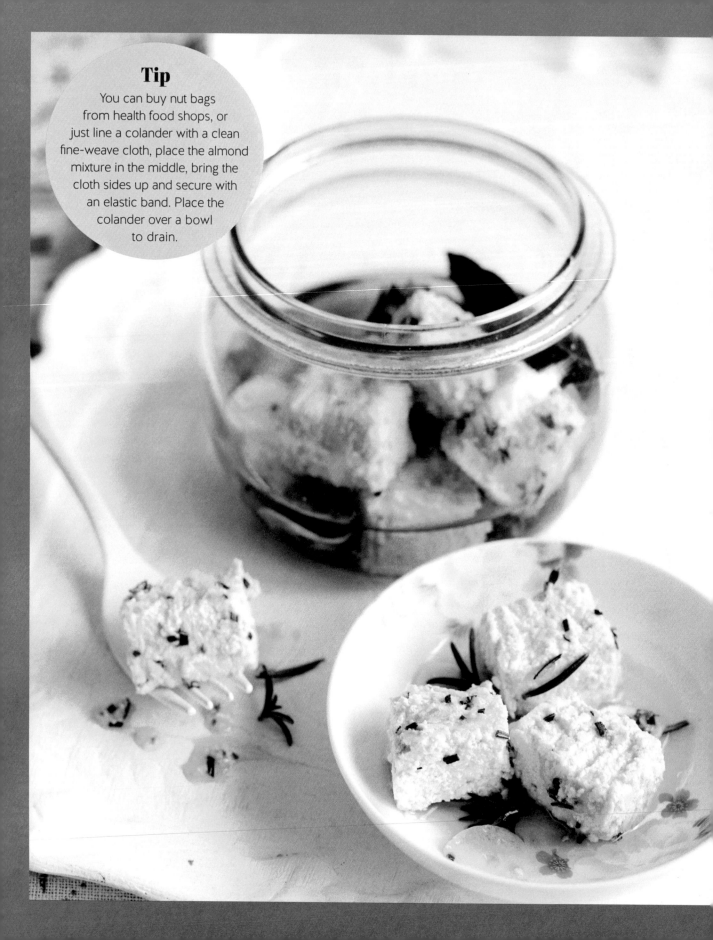

Tip

You can buy nut bags
from health food shops, or
just line a colander with a clean
fine-weave cloth, place the almond
mixture in the middle, bring the
cloth sides up and secure with
an elastic band. Place the
colander over a bowl
to drain.

Rosemary and Garlic Marinated Almond Feta

Little beats the simple trio of olive oil, garlic and salt. The rosemary adds a classic herby punch to this creamy, lemon-scented almond feta. Serve on top of salads, or with crusty bread as part of an antipasto platter.

1 cup blanched almonds
¼ cup lemon juice
1 tablespoon olive oil
1 teaspoon salt

ROSEMARY AND GARLIC MARINADE

1½ cups good-quality extra
    virgin olive oil
1–2 large garlic cloves, crushed
4 tablespoons roughly chopped
    rosemary leaves

- Put the almonds, lemon juice, olive oil and salt in a high-powered blender or food processor. The almonds can be soaked for a few hours before blending, to soften them. Add ½ cup water and blend together for about 5 minutes, until smooth.

- Place the mixture in a nut bag. Place your hands at the top of the bag, above the mixture, squeeze together tightly, then secure the bag with an elastic band. Place in a colander, setting it over a bowl so any excess liquid can drain into the bowl. Refrigerate overnight.

- The next day, carefully remove the almond feta from the nut bag. Discard the draining water. Put the feta in a small square container. Press it down so that it takes on the square shape, and place it back in the fridge for about 30 minutes to set.

- Mix the marinade ingredients together really well. Season to taste with salt, then pour into a shallow serving bowl.

- Carefully turn the feta out onto a chopping board and cut it into small squares. It is super soft like Persian feta, so it breaks easily. Place the squares into the marinade and serve.

Recipe contributed by Melanie Baker, The Kind Cook

Cashew Parmesan

A healthier alternative to parmesan, and 100% kind to cows, this cashew creation lasts for several weeks in the fridge. It tastes great as a cheesy hit on top of pastas, bakes, pizzas, bruschetta and more. If you can't get your hands on cashews, try using raw almonds or pine nuts instead.

1 cup raw cashews
¼ cup nutritional yeast
1 teaspoon salt
½ teaspoon garlic powder

- Put all the ingredients in a food processor. Blend until the nuts are finely ground and the ingredients are well mixed.

- Store in a clean jar in the fridge and use within a few weeks.

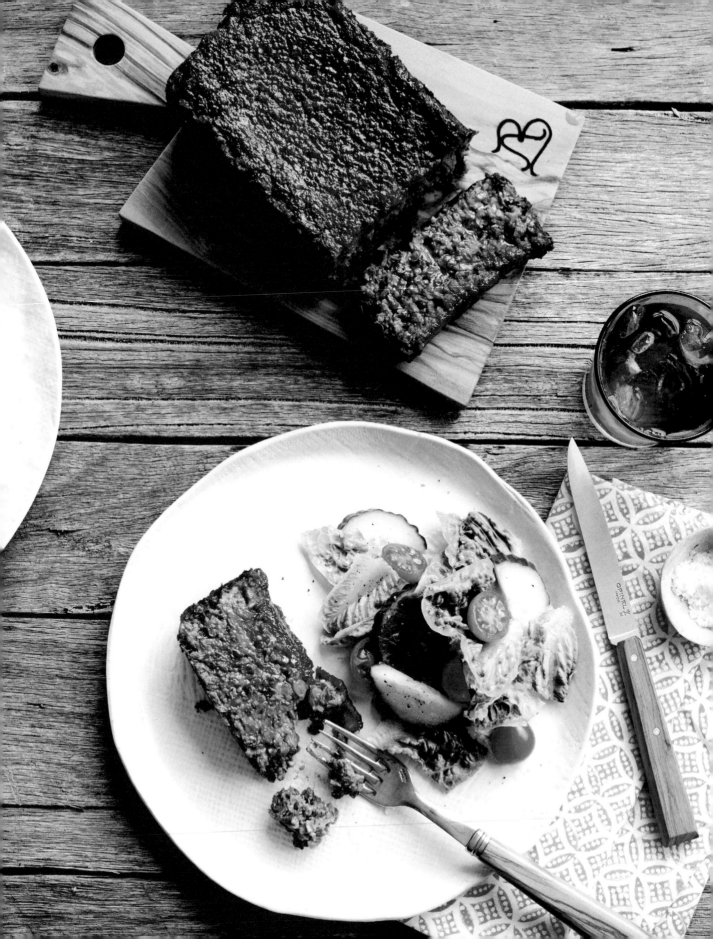

Epic Vegie Loaf with Tomato and Chilli Glaze

SERVES 4

*When you're craving something warm and hearty, this tasty loaf with a sweet
and spicy glaze makes for a perfect winter feed served with roast spuds and vegies.
It also tastes great reheated as leftovers the next day – if there are any!*

1 cup puy lentils

1 cup pecans

3 carrots, roughly chopped

1 large brown onion, roughly chopped

2 garlic cloves, chopped

1–2 tablespoons olive oil

¼ cup raisins or sultanas

1 teaspoon curry powder

½ teaspoon chilli powder

2–3 tablespoons ground flaxseeds

1–2 tablespoons chia seeds

2–3 tablespoons apple sauce

1 tablespoon peanut butter

¼ cup warm water

1 cup finely chopped string beans

Himalayan salt, to taste

TOMATO, CHILLI & GARLIC GLAZE

1 cup tomato sauce

1 teaspoon smoked paprika

½ teaspoon garlic powder
   or granules

a dash of olive oil

¼ cup warm water

30 ml sweet chilli sauce

- Put the lentils in a saucepan, cover with plenty of cold water and bring to the boil. Reduce the heat and gently simmer for 20–30 minutes, or until tender. Drain and set aside.

- Meanwhile, put the pecans in a food processor and blitz for a few seconds. Add the carrots, onion and garlic and process for another few seconds.

- Heat the olive oil in a wide shallow saucepan over medium heat. Add the mixture from the food processor and cook, stirring, for a few minutes, until the onions are translucent and soft; keep an eye on the mixture so it doesn't burn.

- Stir in the raisins, spices and seeds, then the apple sauce, peanut butter and warm water. Add the beans, then stir in the drained lentils. Season to taste with salt and cook, stirring, for about 10 minutes, to bring all the flavours together.

- Meanwhile, preheat the oven to 200°C conventional, or 180°C fan-forced. Grease a 25 cm x 15 cm loaf tin and line it with baking paper.

- Allow the lentil mixture to cool slightly, then roughly mash it, so that it has some texture but is a little on the mushy side too. (If you prefer, you can blend about one-quarter of the mixture in a food processor, then stir it back into the remaining unprocessed mixture.)

- Spoon the lentil mixture into the loaf tin, pressing it down with a spatula, so that it is flat on top.

- In a large mug or glass bowl, thoroughly mix all the glaze ingredients together. Spread the glaze evenly over the top of the loaf.

- Bake for 1 hour, or until the edges are golden.

- In summer serve with a simple coleslaw and green salad, or in winter with a baked potato and steamed vegies.

Recipe contributed by Miriam Sorrell – Mouthwatering Vegan

Pesto Pasta Bake

SERVES 4-6

You know when you make extra food so there'll be leftovers the next day, but then somehow there aren't any? This is that dish! We're not sure if it's the pasta, the basil or the cheesy béchamel, but prepare yourself for firsts, seconds and thirds ... preferably on the couch, in your slippers, surrounded by loved ones! A big bowl of this creamy bake is the perfect thing to warm you up when the cold nights roll in.

500 g penne or fusilli pasta
1 tablespoon olive oil
200 g button mushrooms, quartered
1 garlic clove, crushed
150 g baby spinach leaves
¼ cup semi-dried tomatoes
100 g dairy-free cheese,
   grated (optional)
¼ cup breadcrumbs

PESTO

1½ cups basil leaves
2 garlic cloves
⅓ cup pine nuts
⅓ cup extra virgin olive oil (see tip)
1 teaspoon sea salt
3 tablespoons nutritional
   yeast (optional)

BÉCHAMEL SAUCE

3 tablespoons dairy-free margarine
3 tablespoons plain flour
2½ cups soy milk or other
   dairy-free milk

- Preheat the oven to 180°C conventional, or 160°C fan-forced.

- Bring a large saucepan of water to the boil, add the pasta and cook according to the packet instructions. Drain well, then pour into a 30 cm x 20 cm baking dish.

- Meanwhile, heat the olive oil in a frying pan over medium heat. Fry the mushrooms and garlic for about 5 minutes, until soft. Remove from the heat.

- Put all the pesto ingredients in a blender or food processer and blend until smooth, then set aside.

- To make the béchamel sauce, melt the dairy-free margarine in a saucepan over low heat. Stir in the flour until well combined, then gradually add the milk, stirring continuously until a creamy consistency is achieved. Add the pesto and stir until heated through. Season with salt and pepper to taste.

- Add the mushrooms, spinach and tomatoes to the pasta and mix through well. Coat the pasta mixture with the creamy pesto sauce. Top with dairy-free cheese, if using, and sprinkle with the breadcrumbs.

- Bake for 30–40 minutes, or until the sauce is golden and bubbling. Serve hot.

Tip
For a lighter, oil-free pesto, use water instead of the olive oil.

Lentil Shepherd's Pie

SERVES 4-6

Here's a recipe that both shepherds and sheep will love. Traditional flavours, from a recipe that has been passed down for generations, are combined with lentils and chunky vegies to create a nostalgia-inducing, cruelty-free comfort dish that will hit the spot time and time again.

1 tablespoon vegetable oil

1 large brown onion, finely diced

2–3 large garlic cloves, crushed

2 large unpeeled carrots, grated (to make 2 cups)

4 celery stalks, finely sliced (to make 2 cups)

1 teaspoon hot chilli powder

1 tablespoon ground cumin

2 teaspoons ground coriander

2 tablespoons curry powder

1½ cups green or brown lentils (see tip), rinsed well

400 g tin crushed tomatoes

5 cups vegan beef-style stock

6 mashing potatoes, peeled and diced (to make 6 cups)

¼ cup dairy-free milk, such as almond or rice milk

- Gently heat the oil in a large saucepan and sauté the onion over medium heat for about 5 minutes, or until softened. Add the garlic and stir for another minute or two. Add the carrot and celery and cook for another 5 minutes.

- Meanwhile, in a small frying pan, dry roast the spices over low heat, stirring frequently for a minute or two to bring out their fragrance. Immediately remove from the heat, so the spices don't burn.

- Stir the spices into the sautéed vegetables, along with the lentils, tomatoes and stock. Bring to the boil, then turn the heat down to a very gentle simmer. Cook the lentils, uncovered, for 45 minutes, or until tender. During this time, you can add a little extra stock if you need to, but you don't want the lentils to be too watery, or the mashed potato will just fall into them.

- While the lentils are cooking, bring a large saucepan of water to the boil. Add the potatoes and cook for 10–15 minutes, or until tender; the smaller the cubes the faster they will cook. Drain the potatoes, then add the milk and mash together to a nice smooth piping consistency, adding a little extra milk if you need to. Season well with salt and pepper to taste.

- Meanwhile, preheat the oven to 200°C conventional, or 180°C fan-forced.

- Once the lentils are cooked, place them in a baking dish and allow them to cool a little.

- Attach a large piping nozzle to a piping bag and spoon some mashed potato into it. The mash needs to be quite hot to pipe well, so wrap a tea towel around the piping bag so you can hold it without burning yourself. Pipe rosettes onto the lentils until they are all covered.

- Pop the baking dish in the oven and bake for about 15 minutes, or until the potato topping starts to brown.

- Remove from the oven and leave to set for a few minutes before serving.

Tip

Different varieties of lentils cook at different rates. Check the cooking instructions on the packet, as this will affect how much stock you need, as well as the overall flavour of the final dish.

Recipe contributed by Melanie Baker, The Kind Cook

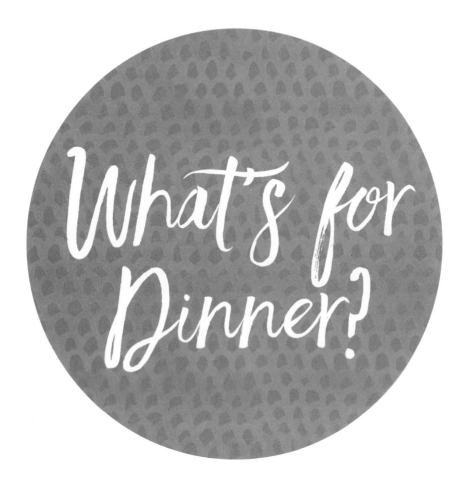

What's for Dinner?

Bring a whole world of compassionate cooking into your dining room every night of the week. From noodle dishes and curries, to pies, stews and stir-fries, these hearty mains are as good for you as they are kind to animals and the planet.

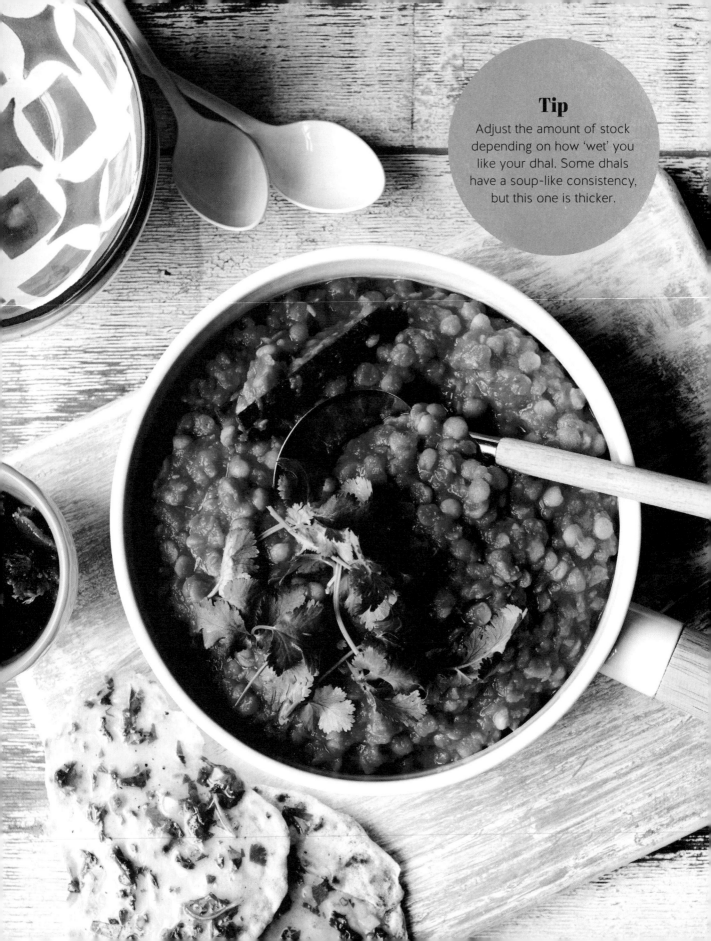

Tip

Adjust the amount of stock depending on how 'wet' you like your dhal. Some dhals have a soup-like consistency, but this one is thicker.

Yellow Split Pea Dhal with Garlic Naan

SERVES 4-6

Yellow split peas are delicious in this dhal, but you can use other pulses such as red lentils, chickpeas or split chickpeas; adjust the cooking time accordingly, as red lentils will cook more quickly. This curry is quite mild, so add more chilli powder for a hotter dhal, or leave it out.

2 tablespoons coconut oil

1 brown onion

5 cardamom pods, lightly pounded

1 cinnamon stick

1½ teaspoons cumin seeds

4 garlic cloves, crushed

5 cm piece fresh ginger,
   peeled and grated

½ teaspoon ground turmeric

3 teaspoons ground coriander

1 teaspoon curry powder

¼ teaspoon chilli powder, or to taste

1¼ cups dried yellow split peas,
   rinsed well

400 g tin whole peeled tomatoes

2-3 cups vegetable stock (see tip)

1 teaspoon lemon juice

½ bunch coriander, chopped

GARLIC NAAN

1 tablespoon dairy-free margarine

2 garlic cloves, crushed

1 cup coriander leaves, washed,
   then finely chopped

2 cups plain flour

1 teaspoon salt

1 teaspoon baking powder

¼ cup soy milk

2 tablespoons extra virgin olive oil

- Heat the coconut oil in a large non-stick saucepan and sauté the onion over low heat for about 10 minutes, or until soft. Add the cardamom pods and cinnamon stick and stir for 1 minute, then stir in the cumin seeds. Add the garlic, ginger and a pinch of salt and mix together. Add the turmeric, ground coriander, curry and chilli powders and stir for a further 1-2 minutes, until the spices release their flavour.

- Now add the split peas and cook, stirring frequently, for 3-5 minutes, taking care not to let them stick to the pan. Stir in the tomatoes and vegetable stock until well combined, then bring to a simmer. Cook, uncovered, for 30 minutes, or until the split peas are soft, adding a little more stock or water if needed.

- While the split peas are simmering, make the garlic naan. Melt the margarine in a small non-stick saucepan over medium heat and fry the garlic and coriander for about 30 seconds, until the garlic becomes aromatic. Set aside.

- Combine the remaining naan ingredients in a bowl, pour in ½ cup water and mix into a soft dough using your hands, adding more flour if needed to bring the dough together. Knead the dough gently in the bowl until soft and supple.

- Break the dough into 8-10 smaller balls. On a flour-dusted work surface, roll out each ball into a flat circle about 5 mm thick, stacking them between sheets of baking paper so they don't stick together.

- Heat a non-stick frying pan over medium-high heat. Place one of the dough circles in the pan; bubbles will start to form. After 1-2 minutes, flip the naan over and cook the other side for a further 1-2 minutes, until golden brown in patches. Remove from the pan and place on a sheet of foil. Lightly brush with the sautéed garlic mixture, sprinkle with a pinch of salt, then close the foil over the naan to keep it warm.

- Cook the remaining naan breads in the same way. You can keep them warm in a low oven (100-120°C), wrapped in foil, until ready to serve.

- Just before serving, stir the lemon juice and coriander leaves through the dhal. Serve with the warm naan breads.

Salt and Pepper Tofu

SERVES 4

These crispy golden nuggets are spicy and aromatic, and pair perfectly with simple steamed rice or quinoa and a side of Sesame soy seasonal greens (page 215) for a quick mid-week meal.

300 g firm tofu
1 teaspoon salt
1½ tablespoons cornflour
2 tablespoons rice bran oil
2 teaspoons sesame oil
1 tablespoon finely grated fresh ginger
    or galangal
1 celery stalk, with small leaves, diced
4 spring onions, thinly sliced, plus
    extra to garnish
1 dried red chilli, crumbled (optional)
2 garlic cloves, very finely sliced
1–1½ teaspoons black pepper, to taste
2 teaspoons soy sauce or tamari
1 teaspoon sushi seasoning or rice
    wine vinegar (see tip)
lemon wedges, to serve

- Cut the tofu into bite-sized pieces and place in a heatproof bowl. Sprinkle with the salt, then cover with boiling water. Leave to tenderise for 10–15 minutes, then drain and pat dry with a clean tea towel. Place in a bowl and toss with the cornflour, coating each piece of tofu.

- Heat the rice bran and sesame oils in a large frying pan over medium-high heat. Fry the tofu pieces for about 5 minutes on each side, until golden brown and crispy. Remove with tongs or a slotted spoon and drain on paper towel, leaving as much oil in the pan as you can.

- To the same frying pan, add the ginger, celery, spring onions and chilli, if using. Sauté for about 1 minute, stirring frequently, until the spring onions have softened. Add the garlic and cook for a further 20 seconds, until aromatic. Stir in the black pepper until well combined, then sprinkle in the soy sauce.

- Immediately tip the tofu back into the pan and toss well to coat with the spices. Add the sushi seasoning, stir one last time, then remove from the heat.

- Plate up, then garnish with extra spring onions. Serve with lemon wedges on the side.

Tip

Adding a splash of vinegar at the end of cooking really helps boost the flavours of foods. It bumps up the freshness and complexity of the dish, without the need to add extra salt.

Lemony Risotto with Seasonal Greens

SERVES 4 GENEROUSLY, WITH ENOUGH LEFT TO MAKE RISOTTO CAKES THE NEXT DAY

The idea of making risotto can be a little daunting, but the truth is it's not difficult. The whole stirring process can actually be quite soothing on a lazy Sunday evening – one glass of wine for the rice, one for you … Fresh lemon and mint provide a burst of summer flavour, even in the depths of winter. Arborio rice is quite creamy without the addition of dairy, and this recipe really lets the sweetness of your chosen vegies shine through. Using a wide, heavy-based cast-iron pan will help spread the heat and cook the risotto evenly.

2 litres vegetable stock

250 g fresh seasonal greens, such as asparagus, cut into bite-sized pieces

2 cups broad beans, double-shelled (see tip)

1½ cups baby peas, fresh or frozen

⅓ cup olive oil

1 leek, pale section only, halved lengthways and thoroughly cleaned of grit, then thinly sliced

1 garlic clove, crushed

500 g arborio rice

100 ml dry white wine

zest and juice of 1 lemon

⅓ cup shredded mint leaves, plus extra mint sprigs to garnish

Cashew parmesan (page 187) or nutritional yeast, to serve (optional)

Tip

Frozen broad beans are easier to shell than fresh. Place in a bowl and cover with boiling water. When cool enough to handle, simply pop the tender, bright green inner beans out of their tough outer shells.

- In a large saucepan, heat the vegetable stock to simmering point. Add the asparagus, broad beans and peas and blanch for about 30 seconds in the hot stock; remove using tongs or a sieve, quickly refresh in cold water and set aside. Keep the stock at a simmer.

- Heat a separate heavy cast-iron pan or deep frying pan over medium–low heat. Add the olive oil and allow to warm for about 1 minute before adding the leek. Sauté for about 5 minutes, or until the leek is soft, then add the garlic and stir constantly for 20 seconds. Pour in the rice and mix to thoroughly coat with the leek-infused oil. Continue stirring constantly until the rice starts to look translucent – be careful not to let it brown! Add the wine and stir until it is mostly all absorbed. Now, pour yourself a glass of wine and get ready to stir.

- One at a time, add ladlefuls of the simmering stock to the rice, stirring until the stock has been absorbed before adding more. Continue this process until the rice is cooked to your liking – some people prefer it *al dente* with a little bite, others like it smooshier (just don't let risotto purists see it!). This could take up to 40 minutes, so make sure you're wearing comfy shoes and the wine is within reach …

- Finally, stir in the lemon zest, lemon juice and shredded mint, along with your blanched asparagus, broad beans and peas; allow the vegies to warm through. Season to taste with salt and pepper before ladling into warmed serving bowls. Garnish with mint sprigs and serve with cashew parmesan or nutritional yeast for sprinkling over if desired.

Variations

- In winter, instead of asparagus, sauté some kale or cavolo nero with a crushed garlic clove in a little olive oil. Season to taste with salt and pepper and spoon over the cooked risotto just before serving. You may also like to replace the mint with parsley or some basil.

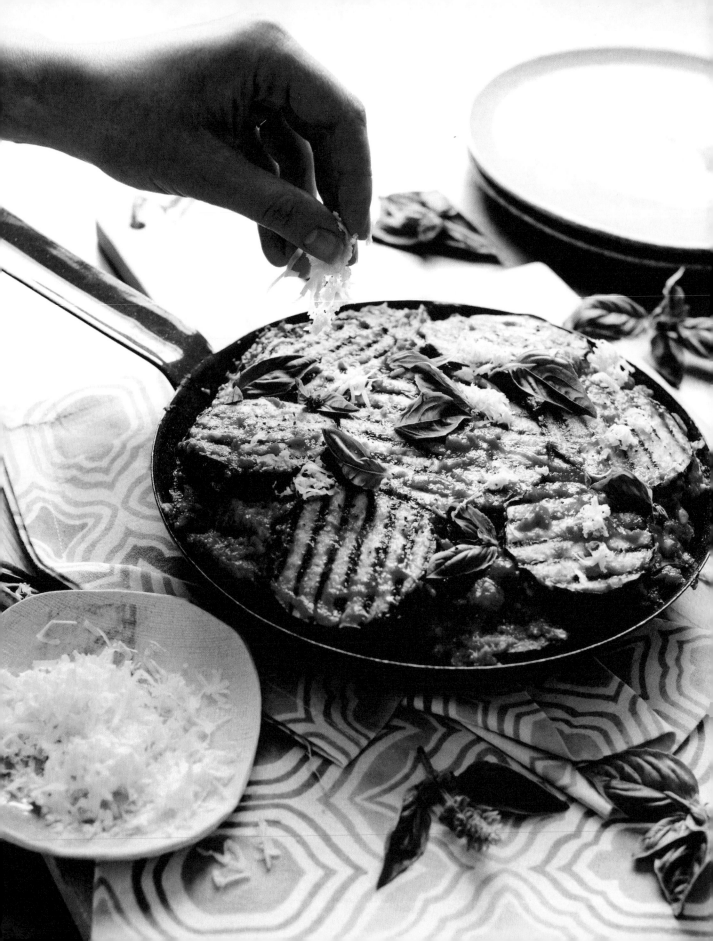

Layered Cheesy Eggplant Bake

SERVES 4

This lightened-up version of the classic Italian dish aubergine parmigiana is made with tender, smoky grilled eggplant slices, layered with breadcrumbs and a rich tomato sauce. Serve hot, cut into wedges, with a crisp green salad and a carafe of vino … Salute to that!

½ cup olive oil

1 large onion, finely chopped

2–3 garlic cloves, crushed

1 teaspoon dried oregano

½ teaspoon dried sage

1 tablespoon tomato paste

a pinch of sugar

2 tablespoons red wine or
    dry marsala

750 g jar of tomato passata

½–1 cup vegetable stock (or water)

4 medium-sized eggplants (about
    700–800 g in total)

75–100 g dairy-free cheese, either
    cut into slices or grated, plus extra
    to garnish

⅓ cup basil leaves, plus extra
    to garnish

1 cup panko breadcrumbs (mixed
    with 1 tablespoon nutritional yeast,
    optional)

FOR TOPPING

1 cup panko breadcrumbs

2 tablespoons olive oil

- Warm half the olive oil in a large heavy-based saucepan over medium heat. Add the onion and sauté, stirring occasionally, for about 8 minutes, until golden brown and softened. Add the garlic and dried herbs, and cook for a further 30 seconds, until fragrant. Stir in the tomato paste and sugar. Cook for another minute, until the sugar has dissolved, and the tomato paste turns a slightly darker red. Deglaze the pan with the wine or marsala, stirring for about 1 minute to allow the alcohol to evaporate.

- Stir in the passata. Bring to the boil, stirring constantly, then immediately reduce the heat to low. Cover and leave to simmer for 10 minutes, stirring occasionally so the sauce doesn't stick. Add the stock and mix well. Remove from the heat, season to taste and set aside.

- While the sauce is simmering, prepare the eggplants. Heat your barbecue to medium–high; alternatively, use a chargrill pan. Trim the ends from each eggplant, then slice lengthways into 1 cm strips. Lightly brush each side of the eggplant with the remaining olive oil, then grill in batches for about 5 minutes on each side, or until slightly charred and tender enough for a knife to pierce the middle easily.

- Preheat the oven to 200°C conventional, or 180°C fan-forced. Lightly grease a 25 cm round baking dish.

- Ladle one-quarter of the tomato sauce mixture over the bottom of the dish, then add enough eggplant slices to cover in a single layer. Sprinkle with one-third of the cheese, a few basil leaves and one-third of the breadcrumbs. Continue layering with the tomato sauce, eggplant, cheese, basil and breadcrumbs until you've used up all your eggplant – make sure your second-last layer is tomato sauce!

- Sprinkle with the topping breadcrumbs to create a crust. Drizzle with the olive oil and pop the whole thing in the oven.

- Bake for 25–30 minutes, until the breadcrumb crust is lightly golden. Remove from the oven and leave to stand for a few minutes to let the layers fuse; it will be molten hot!

- Use a very sharp knife to cut the eggplant bake into wedges. Garnish with extra cheese and basil leaves and tuck in.

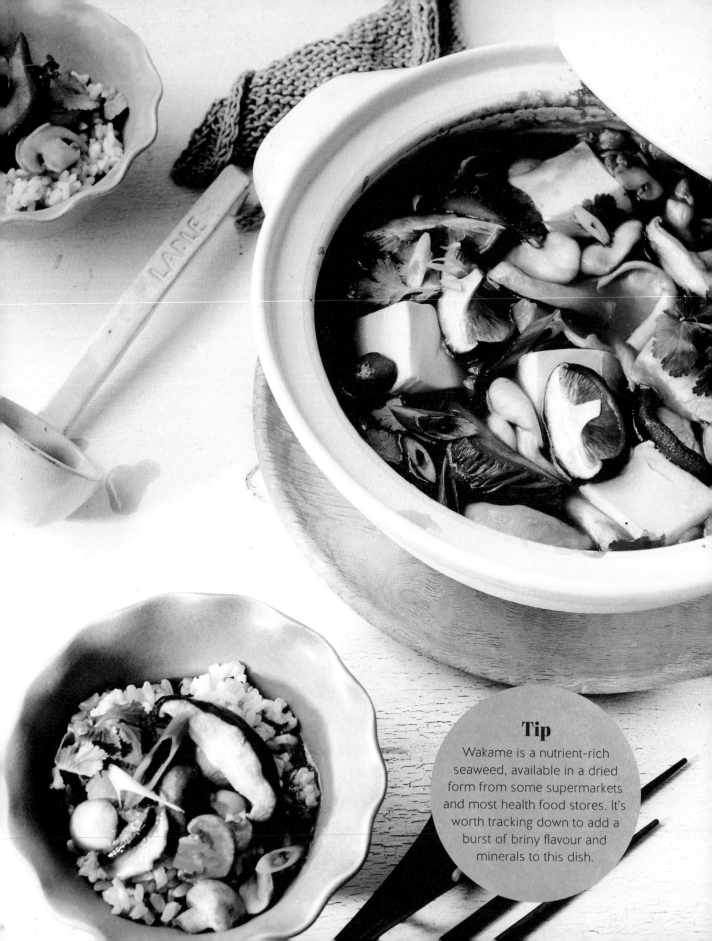

Tip

Wakame is a nutrient-rich seaweed, available in a dried form from some supermarkets and most health food stores. It's worth tracking down to add a burst of briny flavour and minerals to this dish.

Chinese Mushroom Hot Pot

SERVES 4

A rich, hearty stew that's perfect for those chilly autumn evenings. Serve with white or brown rice, quinoa or millet to soak up all the lovely gravy. Experiment with a variety of mushrooms for flavour and texture – you might find a new favourite!

150 g mixed mushrooms, such as fresh shiitake, oyster, shimeji, black fungus or enoki, or tinned straw mushrooms

400 g white button mushrooms

1 tablespoon cornflour

1½ cups vegetable stock

2 tablespoons hoisin sauce

2 tablespoons soy sauce

2–3 tablespoons olive oil

1 teaspoon sesame oil

4 garlic cloves, crushed

½ teaspoon Chinese five-spice powder

1 teaspoon crumbled, dried wakame (optional; see tip)

200 g silken tofu, cut into 2 cm cubes (optional)

snipped coriander, to garnish (optional)

sliced spring onions, to garnish (optional)

- Preheat the oven to 200°C conventional, or 180°C fan-forced. Lightly oil a casserole dish with a lid.

- Brush the mushrooms free of dirt. Cut or tear the fresh mixed mushrooms into bite-sized pieces, keeping the different varieties separate, so they can be added to the hot pot at different stages to maintain their lovely textures. Slice the button mushrooms and set aside. (We'll be adding the sturdier ones first, and saving the more delicate enoki and oyster mushrooms until the very end, so keeping them all separate will make this easier to do.)

- Mix the cornflour to a smooth paste with some of the vegetable stock in a bowl. Add the remaining vegetable stock, then stir in the hoisin and soy sauces until well combined. Set aside.

- In a large saucepan, gently heat the olive and sesame oils over medium heat. Add the garlic and Chinese five-spice and stir for about 20 seconds, until aromatic.

- Now add the button mushrooms, and any fresh shiitake, and stir to coat with the garlicky oil. After about 5 minutes, when they've softened slightly, add any shimeji mushrooms or black fungus, and any tinned straw mushrooms. Cook, stirring frequently, for 1 minute.

- Give the vegetable stock mixture a quick stir, then pour over the mushrooms, stirring constantly. Bring the mixture to a low boil, stirring constantly for 3–4 minutes, until the sauce has thickened slightly.

- Stir in any oyster mushrooms, and the wakame, if using. Pour the mixture into your casserole dish. Arrange any enoki mushrooms on top, and the silken tofu, if using, poking the cubes down into the hot pot slightly.

- Pop the lid on, transfer to the oven and bake for 20 minutes. Check to see if the mushrooms are cooked to your liking, and add a little more vegetable stock or water if the hot pot looks a little dry. Cover and bake for a further 10–15 minutes, if required.

- Remove from the oven and leave to sit for 10 minutes. Garnish with coriander or spring onions (or both!) and serve with steamed rice, quinoa or millet.

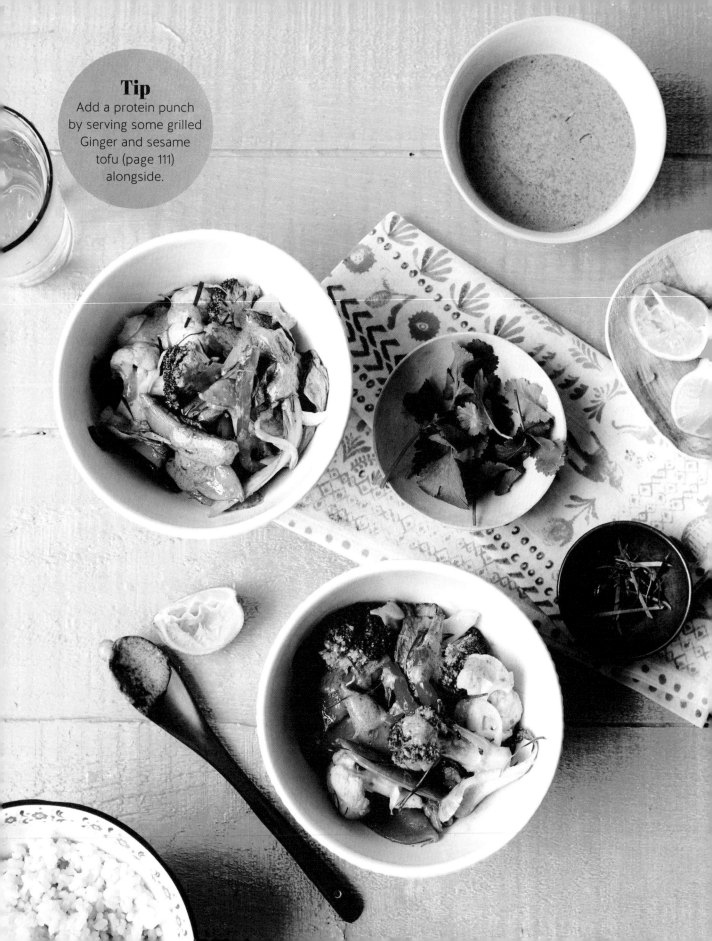

Tip
Add a protein punch
by serving some grilled
Ginger and sesame
tofu (page 111)
alongside.

Vegie Stir-fry with Coconut Red Curry Sauce

SERVES 4

There are no hard and fast rules here. Feel free to choose your favourite rainbow-mix of ingredients; just be sure to add more robust vegies such as cauliflower and carrot early, and delicate ones like snow peas in the last minute or so of cooking. The other trick to a good stir-fry is to make sure your vegies are dry before adding them to the hot pan, otherwise they'll steam and lose their fresh, crisp texture. Serve with steamed brown rice or noodles for a quick mid-week meal.

2 teaspoons rice bran oil

1 teaspoon sesame oil

½ cauliflower, cut into bite-sized florets

1 carrot, julienned or very thinly sliced

1 head of broccoli, cut into
   bite-sized florets

6–8 cups delicate greens (such as
   wombok cabbage or bok choy),
   cut into 3 cm pieces

½ red capsicum, seeded and cut into
   thick slices

1 teaspoon finely grated fresh ginger

zest of ½ lemon

200 g snow peas or sugar snap peas

1 teaspoon rice wine vinegar or apple
   cider vinegar

⅓ cup roughly chopped coriander
   (optional)

4 kaffir lime leaves, very finely
   shredded, to garnish (optional)

1 lemon or lime, cut into wedges,
   to serve

RED CURRY SAUCE

1 tablespoon vegan red curry paste

1 cup coconut milk

½ cup vegetable stock (or water)

4–6 kaffir lime leaves, very
   finely shredded

juice of 1 lemon

• To make the red curry sauce, warm a heavy-based saucepan over medium heat, then add the curry paste. Let it fry, stirring occasionally, for 1 minute, before adding ½ cup of the coconut milk. Stir well, then let the mixture simmer and reduce for about 5 minutes, stirring occasionally to make sure it doesn't stick.

• Add the remaining coconut milk, the stock and lime leaves, and mix well. Reduce the heat to a low simmer and let the sauce bubble away and thicken while you prepare the vegies. Just before you are ready to serve, stir in the lemon juice.

• Heat a wok over medium-high heat. When it is hot, add the rice bran and sesame oils. Add the cauliflower and carrot and cook for about 2 minutes, stirring constantly to make sure the cauliflower florets cook evenly. Now add the broccoli and continue to stir. When the broccoli, carrot and cauliflower are tender, but not too soft, add the cabbage or bok choy, capsicum, ginger, lemon zest and snow peas. Toss well to combine, and fry for a mere minute or two, until the cabbage is **just** wilted and the peas have turned bright green, but still retain a bit of bite.

• Immediately remove from the heat and sprinkle with the vinegar.

• Serve with steamed brown rice or noodles, drizzled with the red curry sauce, sprinkled with chopped coriander and shredded lime leaves if desired, with a lemon or lime wedge on the side.

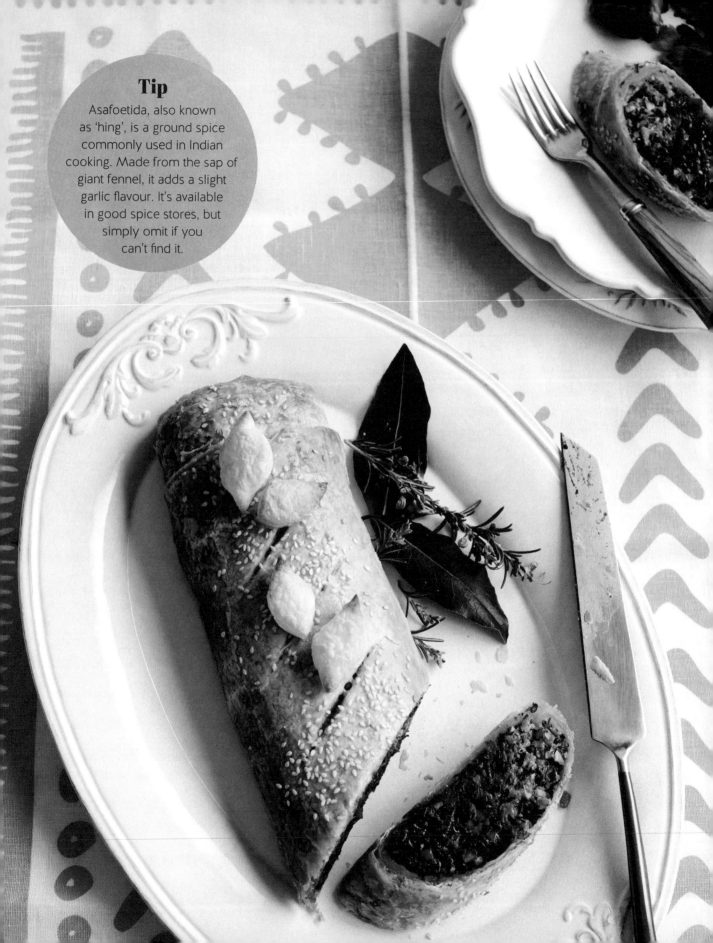

Tip

Asafoetida, also known as 'hing', is a ground spice commonly used in Indian cooking. Made from the sap of giant fennel, it adds a slight garlic flavour. It's available in good spice stores, but simply omit if you can't find it.

Double-stuffed Savoury Festive Log

SERVES 8

Infused with herbs and a touch of spice, this succulent, savoury log is the perfect main course for Christmas, or a Sunday roast with family or friends – it's healthy, decadent and mouthwatering!

3 thawed dairy-free puff pastry sheets

dairy-free milk, for brushing

MUSHROOM AND CURRIED LENTIL STUFFING

1–2 tablespoons extra virgin olive oil

1 brown onion, finely chopped

2 garlic cloves, finely chopped

1½ tablespoons tomato paste

1 teaspoon smoked paprika

1 teaspoon hot curry powder (or
   ½ teaspoon mild curry powder,
   if you don't like it hot)

⅛ teaspoon asafoetida (see tip)

8 medium-sized mushrooms of
   your choice, finely chopped

¾ cup puy lentils, boiled until cooked,
   then drained and set aside

2 tablespoons chopped sundried
   tomatoes

Himalayan salt, to taste

NUT STUFFING

1 onion, roughly chopped

1–2 garlic cloves, roughly chopped

2 tablespoons roughly chopped
   flat-leaf parsley

1–2 tablespoons chopped rosemary

2–3 sage leaves, or ½ teaspoon
   dried sage

200 g roasted hazelnuts

2 tablespoons breadcrumbs

Himalayan salt, to taste

- To make the lentil stuffing, heat the olive oil in a large saucepan over medium heat. Fry the onion and garlic for about 5 minutes, until softened, then add the tomato paste and all the spices. Mix well, then stir in the mushrooms and cook for about 10 minutes, allowing them to yield all their juices. Stir in the lentils, sundried tomatoes and 1½ tablespoons water and cook for a further 10–15 minutes. Season with salt, and leave to cool before stuffing the pastry – the mixture should be no more than lukewarm.

- While the lentils are simmering, make the nut stuffing. Place the onion, garlic and herbs in a food processor and blend until small pieces form. Next, add the hazelnuts and pulse into crumbs. Add the remaining ingredients, then process for 10–20 seconds, until you have a nice crumble mix, but it's not crushed to a pulp. Set aside.

- Preheat the oven to 220°C conventional, or 200°C fan-forced. Line a baking tray with baking paper.

- Place the pastry sheets on a clean, floured work surface, overlapping them to make a long rectangle. Brush a little milk in between the overlapping edges to help them adhere to each other, then roll the pastry sheets together, with the short length facing you. Leaving a generous border of pastry clear along the bottom and both edges, spoon the lentil stuffing mixture onto the bottom pastry sheet, gently spreading the filling into a square shape. In another square shape, directly above the lentil mixture, spread the nut stuffing mixture, again leaving a generous border clear along both pastry edges and the top.

- Now start slowly rolling the bottom pastry edge over the mixture, away from you, until you reach the end – an extra pair of hands can be helpful here. Don't worry if any bits fall out the side; just gently push them back in place. Secure the folded-over pastry in place using toothpicks. Brush the pastry with a little milk. Using a sharp knife, gently score the surface of the pastry to mark equal serving portions.

- Using two large metal spatulas – again another set of hands can be useful here – carefully lift the log onto the baking tray. Transfer to the oven. Bake for 30 minutes, or until the pastry is puffed and golden. Remove from the oven and leave to cool for a few minutes before slicing. Serve warm.

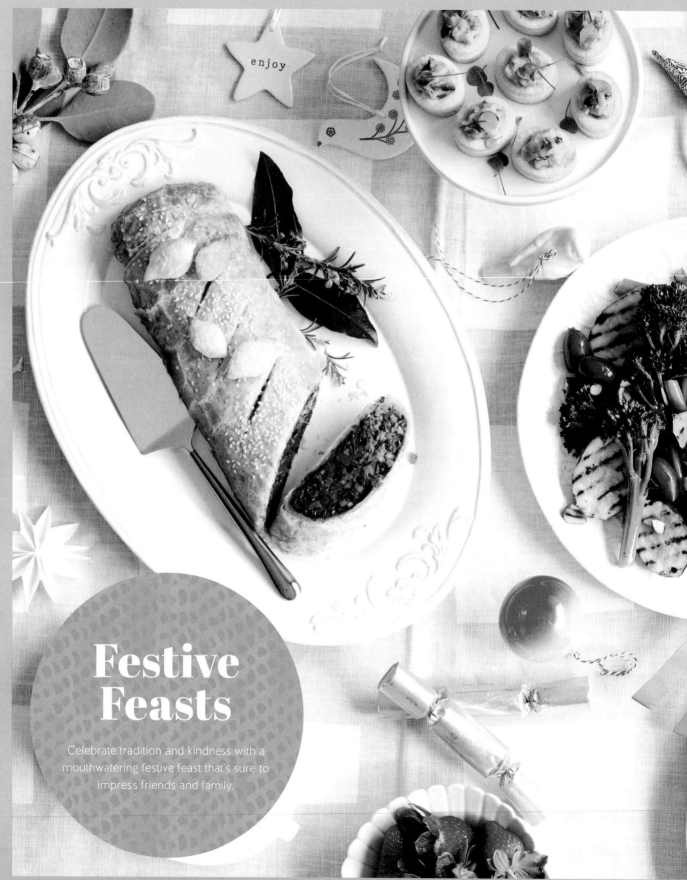

Festive Feasts

Celebrate tradition and kindness with a mouthwatering festive feast that's sure to impress friends and family.

From left to right: Savoury festive log (p 205); Vol-au-vents with garlicky mushroom filling (p 209); Barbecued vegie plate (p 151);

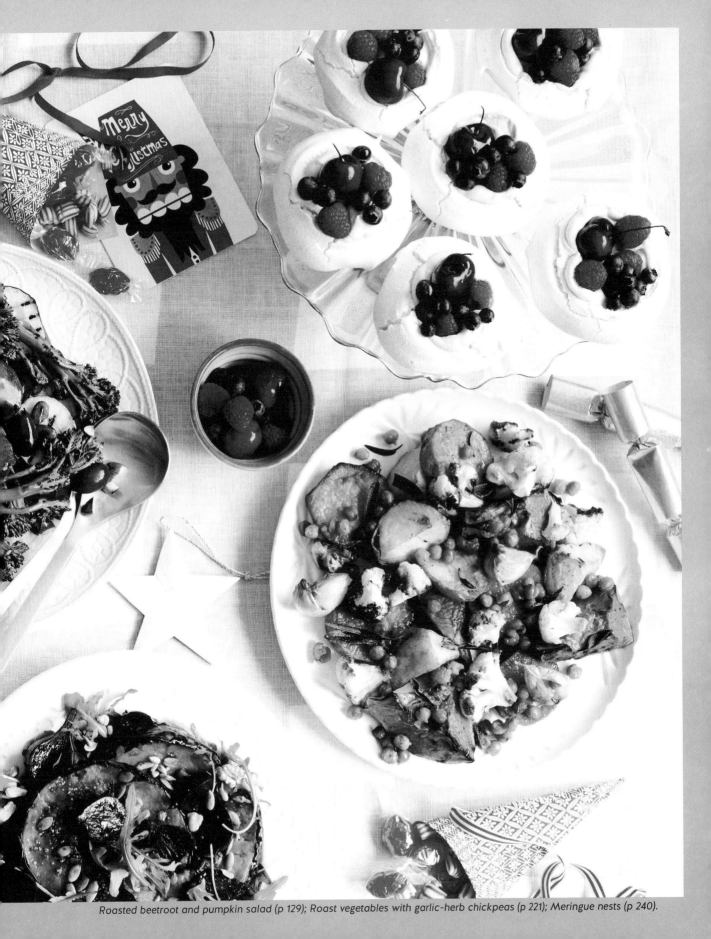

Roasted beetroot and pumpkin salad (p 129); Roast vegetables with garlic-herb chickpeas (p 221); Meringue nests (p 240).

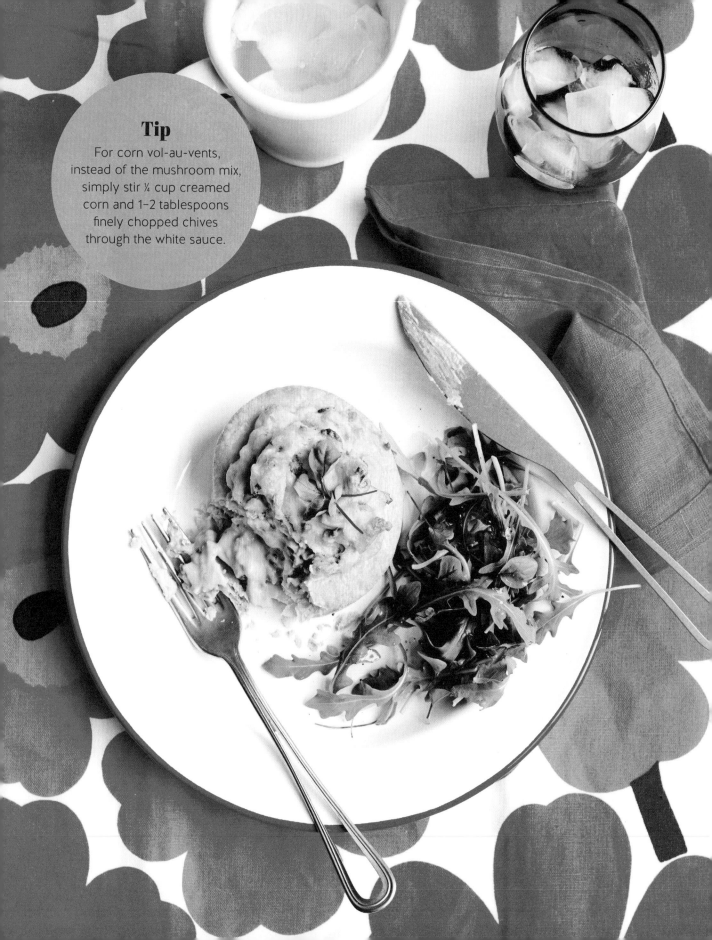

Tip

For corn vol-au-vents,
instead of the mushroom mix,
simply stir ¼ cup creamed
corn and 1–2 tablespoons
finely chopped chives
through the white sauce.

Vol-au-vents with Garlicky Mushroom Filling

SERVES 4

*These crispy bites of golden goodness make an elegant light supper with a side salad.
The filling can be made a day ahead and refrigerated until needed.*

6 sheets of frozen dairy-free
    puff pastry squares, thawed
    but still cold
½ cup soy milk, for brushing
3–4 tablespoons finely
    chopped chives

EASY WHITE SAUCE

¼ cup olive oil
¼ cup chickpea flour (besan)
3 cups full-fat soy milk
3 teaspoons garlic powder
3 teaspoons onion powder
⅓–½ cup nutritional yeast
50 g dairy-free cheese,
    grated (optional)

MUSHROOM MIX

1 tablespoon olive oil
200–300 g button mushrooms,
    some diced, the rest sliced
    (for texture)
1–2 garlic cloves, crushed and
    finely chopped
1 tablespoon finely chopped chives
1 tablespoon roughly chopped
    flat-leaf parsley
⅛ teaspoon freshly grated nutmeg
    (optional)

- Line two baking trays with non-stick baking paper. Cut each square pastry sheet into four even pieces (making 24 pastry squares). Using a round biscuit cutter a little smaller than your pastry squares, cut through the centre of 16 pastry pieces, but leave the pastry in place; this is just so you can lift out the centres after they've cooked to spoon in the filling. Leave eight of the pastry shapes whole to use as the vol-au-vent bases.

- Stack your pastry squares three pieces high, with a whole piece on the bottom, and two cut pieces on top. Brush a little soy milk in between each layer to make them stick. You'll end up with eight vol-au-vent cases. Arrange on the baking trays and chill in the fridge to let the pastry rest.

- To make the white sauce, heat the olive oil in a large saucepan over medium heat. When it is hot, add the chickpea flour, whisking constantly to avoid lumps. Cook, stirring, for about 30 seconds, until the mixture is smooth and the flour starts to smell a little toasty. Gradually add the soy milk, whisking, to form a smooth sauce. Bring to the boil, then immediately reduce the heat to a simmer, stirring constantly until the sauce has thickened. Stir in the garlic and onion powders, then remove from the heat. If the sauce has thickened too much at this point, simply stir in a little more soy milk. Stir in the nutritional yeast and dairy-free cheese, if using. Season to taste with salt and pepper and set aside.

- Preheat the oven to 200°C conventional, or 180°C fan-forced.

- To make the mushroom mix, warm the olive oil in a frying pan over medium heat. Add the mushrooms and cook, stirring occasionally, for about 5 minutes, until soft. Add the garlic and cook for 20 seconds. Remove from the heat and stir in the chives, parsley and nutmeg, if using. Stir the mushroom mix through the white sauce and set aside.

- Brush the tops of your pastry squares with a little soy milk. Transfer to the oven and bake for 20–25 minutes, or until puffed and lightly golden.

- Remove from the oven. When cool enough to handle, use a sharp knife to cut around the circle indentation on the top of your pastry squares and take off their lids. Spoon in the mushroom sauce and sprinkle with half the chopped chives. Bake for a further 10 minutes, or until the filling is heated through and set. Remove from the oven and cool slightly. Serve warm, sprinkled with the remaining chives.

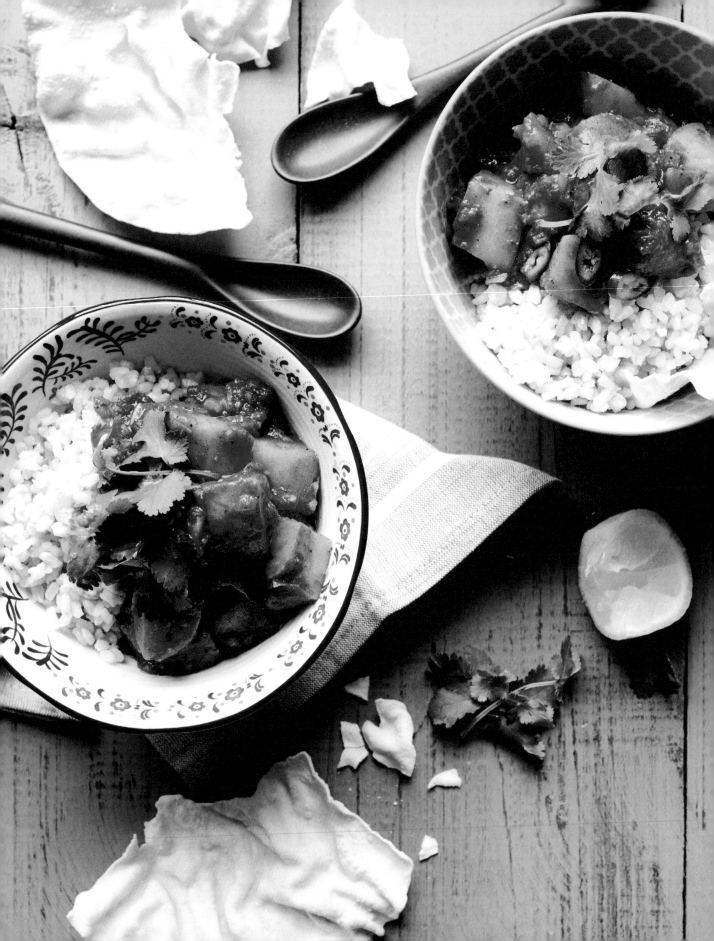

Aloo Curry

SERVES 4

Aloo curry is a tomato-based Indian potato curry, served with roti, rice or papadums … or all three! This recipe is designed for those who like it hot, but you can always tone down the chilli for a milder flavour.

2 tablespoons rice bran
　or grapeseed oil
2 onions, chopped
4 garlic cloves, crushed
3 cm piece fresh ginger, peeled
　and finely chopped
2 teaspoons salt
1 teaspoon ground turmeric
1 teaspoon black pepper
1 teaspoon sweet paprika
1 teaspoon chilli powder
2 teaspoons garam masala
2 tomatoes, peeled, seeded
　and chopped
1 green chilli (or to taste),
　finely chopped
3 large potatoes, peeled (if desired)
　and diced
1 cup fresh or frozen peas (optional)
2 tablespoons coriander leaves,
　to garnish

- Heat the oil in a large heavy-based saucepan. Add the onions and stir constantly over medium–high heat for about 5 minutes, until lightly browned. Add the garlic and ginger and stir constantly until the mixture is lightly golden.

- Add the salt, turmeric, pepper, paprika, chilli powder and garam masala and stir until the spices release their aromas.

- Now add the tomatoes and green chilli and stir constantly for 3–5 minutes, until the tomatoes begin to break down a little. Add the potatoes and stir for another 2 minutes.

- Pour in 1 cup water and stir until well mixed in; if the potatoes aren't covered in liquid, add a little more water. Bring to the boil, then reduce the heat to very low. Put the lid on and simmer for 10–15 minutes, or until the potatoes are tender, stirring often to ensure the mixture doesn't stick to the bottom of the pan.

- When the potatoes are tender, add the peas, if using, then simmer, uncovered, for a few more minutes, to allow the sauce to thicken and the peas to cook.

- Garnish with the coriander and serve hot, with basmati rice, roti or papadums.

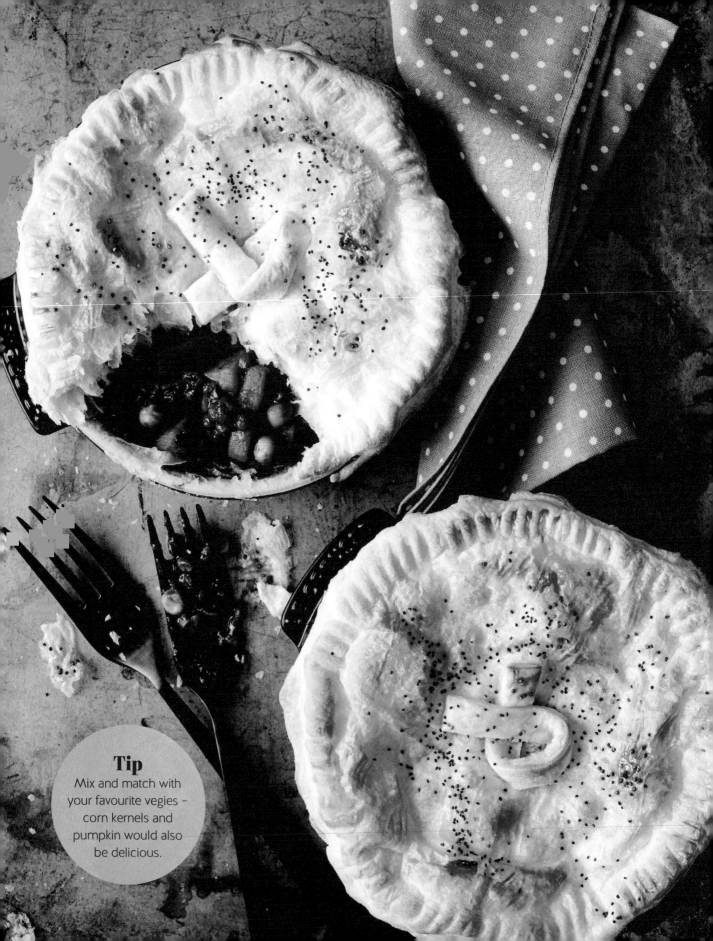

Tip
Mix and match with your favourite vegies – corn kernels and pumpkin would also be delicious.

Double-potato, Mushroom and Lentil Pot Pies

MAKES 4 INDIVIDUAL PIES

Tender, bite-sized pieces of potato, mushroom and carrot nestle in a hearty red wine and thyme lentil gravy. Golden flaky pastry tops it all off – and yes, lashings of tomato sauce are an absolute must. Serve with some simple steamed vegies such as broccolini and cauliflower, sprinkled with a pinch of salt and a splash of apple cider vinegar.

4 sheets of frozen dairy-free puff pastry

2–3 tablespoons olive oil

3 celery stalks, finely diced

2 carrots, halved lenghtways and cut into 5 mm thick half moons

1 large golden onion, finely diced

3–4 large field mushrooms, cut into large wedges or sliced

3 garlic cloves, crushed

1 teaspoon dried sage

1 teaspoon ground coriander

3 thyme sprigs

1 teaspoon finely chopped rosemary

3 waxy potatoes, peeled and cut into 2–3 cm dice

1 small sweet potato, peeled and cut into 1–2 cm dice

1 cup red wine

2 x 400 g tins lentils, drained but not rinsed

2 bay leaves

2½ cups vegan beef-style stock

⅓ cup vegan Worcestershire sauce, to taste

2 tablespoons soy sauce or tamari, to taste

1 heaped tablespoon cornflour or dairy-free instant vegan gravy powder

1 cup fresh or frozen peas

2–3 tablespoons roughly chopped parsley

dairy-free milk, for brushing

- Take your puff pastry out of the freezer and allow to thaw slowly in the fridge while you make the pie filling. Also arrange four ramekins, each 1½–2 cups in capacity, on a baking tray, ready for filling.

- In a large, heavy-based stockpot, warm the olive oil over medium heat. Add the celery, carrots and onion and sauté for about 5 minutes, or until softened. Add the mushrooms and garlic and cook for a further 3–4 minutes, until the mushrooms are tender. Crumble in the dried sage, add the ground coriander and stir well. Add the thyme sprigs, rosemary, potatoes and sweet potato, then give everything a good mix.

- Increase the heat to medium–high and, when the pan is sizzling, pour in the wine. Stir well to deglaze the pan, then let the wine reduce for about 5 minutes. Stir in the lentils, add the bay leaves, then pour in the stock and bring to the boil. Cover the pot, and reduce the heat to a low simmer. Cook, stirring occasionally, for about 30 minutes, until the potatoes are tender.

- Meanwhile, preheat the oven to 240°C conventional, or 220°C fan-forced.

- Stir the Worcestershire and soy sauces through the lentil mixture, along with a few grinds of black pepper. Mix the cornflour or gravy powder to a smooth paste with 2 tablespoons water, then add to the lentils and stir gently for about 1 minute. Remove from the heat and stir in the peas and parsley.

- Discard the bay leaves, then ladle the pie filling evenly into your ramekins. Allow to cool slightly.

- Drape the thawed pastry over the ramekins. Pinch the edges into a decorative pattern, cut a little steam hole in the middle of each and brush the tops with milk.

- Transfer to the oven and bake for 15–20 minutes, or until the filling is bubbling and the pastry is golden brown.

- Remove from the oven and allow to stand for a minute or two before serving.

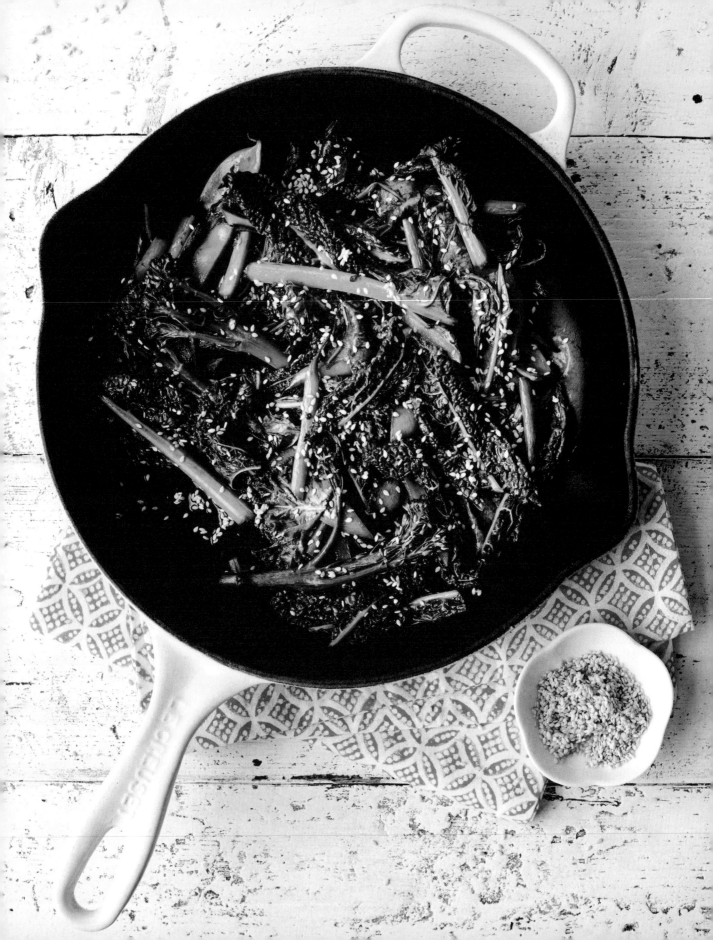

Sesame Soy Seasonal Greens

SERVES 4 AS A SIDE

*We all need to eat our greens; this super quick and simple side dish makes it
a joy, not a chore. Treat your greens right, and they'll treat you good right back.
The trick is to keep them fresh, bright and irresistible, with a bit of a bite.*

1 kg mixed seasonal greens, such as broccoli, English spinach, bok choy, kale, cavolo nero, snow peas, green beans, sugar snap peas, broccolini or pak choy; this sounds like a lot, but leafy greens will reduce considerably during cooking

1 tablespoon rice bran oil

1–2 garlic cloves, crushed

3 cm piece fresh ginger, peeled and finely grated (optional)

1–2 tablespoons soy sauce or tamari

2 tablespoons sesame seeds, toasted (see tip)

2 tablespoons roughly chopped coriander (optional)

- Thoroughly rinse your greens to get rid of any grit. Tear or chop into bite-sized pieces, bearing in mind that tender greens, such as spinach and bok choy, will shrink during cooking.

- If using a mixture of heartier greens like kale, broccoli or cavolo nero, and tender greens like snow peas, place the tougher varieties in a colander and pour boiling water over them until they turn bright green. Immediately blanch under cold running water, then drain. This way they'll cook in the same time as your delicate greens.

- Heat the rice bran oil in a wok or large frying pan over medium heat. Add the garlic and the ginger, if using, and stir constantly for about 20 seconds, until aromatic. Quickly add your greens and, using a spatula or tongs, flip and lift and toss them around so they're covered with the garlic oil and cook evenly. Stir-fry until bright green – this really shouldn't take any longer than 2 minutes.

- Remove from the heat and drizzle with the soy sauce. Serve sprinkled with the toasted sesame seeds, and coriander if desired.

Tip
Use a mix of white and black sesame seeds, if you want to get a little fancy!

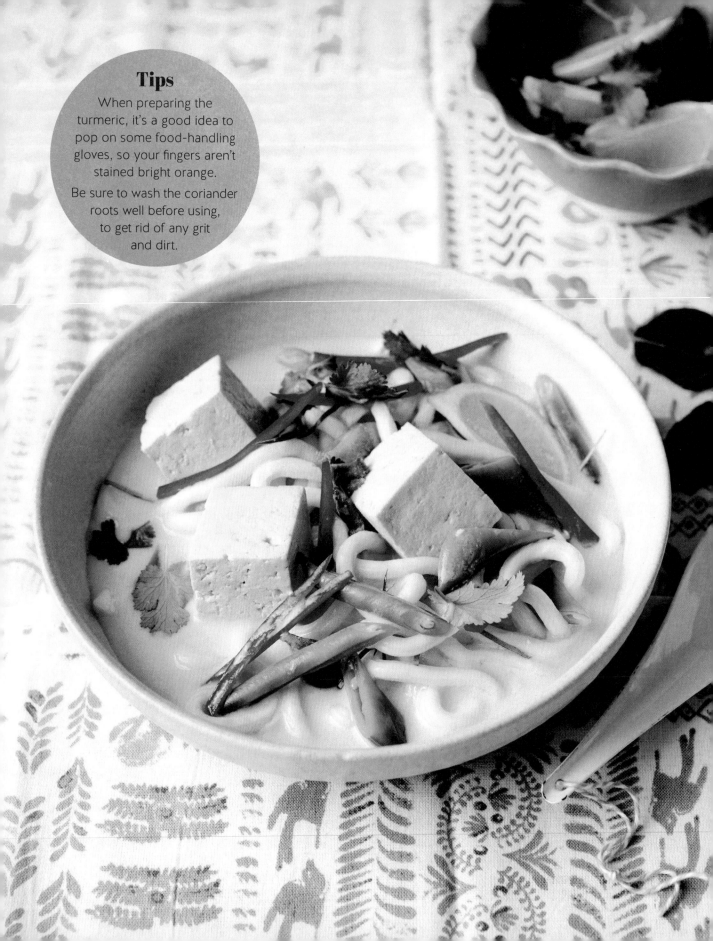

Tips

When preparing the turmeric, it's a good idea to pop on some food-handling gloves, so your fingers aren't stained bright orange.

Be sure to wash the coriander roots well before using, to get rid of any grit and dirt.

Galangal and Tofu Coconut Soup

SERVES 4

Based on a classic Thai soup, this one is full of aromatic herbs and protein-rich tofu, making it both deliciously fragrant and surprisingly hearty.

3½ cups vegan chicken-style stock

3–4 tablespoons peeled and roughly chopped fresh galangal

2–3 cm piece of fresh turmeric, peeled and grated (see tip)

1 lemongrass stem, crushed and roughly chopped

3 tablespoons roughly chopped fresh coriander roots and stems (see tip)

6–8 kaffir lime leaves, torn

450 g firm tofu, thinly sliced

200 g tin straw mushrooms (optional), drained, rinsed and cut in half lengthways

1 red chilli, finely chopped

juice and zest of 2 limes

1 tablespoon grated palm sugar (or brown sugar)

400 ml tin full-cream coconut milk

3–4 tablespoons soy sauce or tamari

1 tablespoon rice wine vinegar (or apple cider vinegar)

400 g soft, wok-ready udon noodles

16 green beans, topped and tailed

16 snow peas or sugar snap peas, topped and tailed

1 small red capsicum, seeded and finely sliced into long strips

2 kaffir lime leaves, very finely shredded, to garnish

4 coriander sprigs, to garnish

1 lime, quartered, to serve

- In a large, heavy-based stockpot, combine the stock, galangal, turmeric, lemongrass, coriander roots and lime leaves. Bring to the boil, then reduce the heat to a gentle simmer for 10 minutes to allow the flavours to infuse. Remove from the heat and leave to stand for 10–20 minutes, before straining into a large jug or bowl. Discard the herbs and spices – they've done their job, leaving you with a gorgeously fragrant soup base.

- Pour the strained soup back into the stockpot and add the tofu and mushrooms, if using. Bring to the boil, then reduce the heat to low and simmer for about 10 minutes, to allow the tofu to absorb all the flavours.

- Stir in the chilli, lime juice, lime zest and palm sugar. Pour in the coconut milk, soy sauce and vinegar, then add the noodles, beans, snow peas and capsicum. Heat, stirring occasionally, until the noodles are separated and warmed through, and the beans are just tender. Be careful not to let the soup boil, or your coconut milk might separate.

- Remove from the heat and ladle into four warmed bowls. Garnish with the shredded lime leaves and coriander sprigs and serve immediately, with lime wedges.

Curried Hokkien Noodles with Tofu

SERVES 4

Bright, aromatic and inescapably – some may say atomically – yellow, this is a variation on Singapore noodles; feel free to use rice vermicelli to make it gluten-free. Now, when stir-frying, there are two things to remember that will make things easier. Firstly, your mise en place: have everything chopped, measured and ready to go next to your stovetop before you put the wok on to heat. Secondly, toss your noodles with the curry powder and seasonings before adding them to the wok – that way you won't risk overcooking them by trying to coat each individual noodle while cooking.

450 g packet fresh hokkien noodles

1 serve of Ginger and sesame tofu (page 111), or a packet of tofu puffs

3 tablespoons grated fresh ginger

4 garlic cloves, crushed

5–6 spring onions, thickly sliced diagonally

1–1½ tablespoons mild curry powder (or use a hot curry powder, if you like it spicy!)

½ x 225 g tin water chestnuts, sliced

8 fresh shiitake mushrooms, sliced

1 carrot, cut into small dice

1 small red capsicum, seeded and cut into thin strips

100 g frozen peas

300 g green beans

100–120 ml soy sauce

⅓ cup mirin or sake

1 teaspoon sugar

2 teaspoons sesame oil

⅓ cup rice bran oil

⅓–½ cup roughly chopped coriander, to garnish

lemon wedges, to serve

- Put the noodles in a heatproof bowl and cover with boiling water. Leave for 3 minutes, then drain in a colander and leave to air dry for about 15 minutes (this way the curry mix will stick to them better).

- While waiting for the noodles to dry, fry your marinated Ginger and sesame tofu in a wok over medium–high heat until lightly browned, then set aside on a plate. If you're using tofu puffs, you can skip this step.

- In a small bowl, mix together the ginger, garlic, spring onions and half the curry powder.

- In another small bowl, combine the water chestnuts, mushrooms, carrot, capsicum and frozen peas.

- Top and tail the green beans, then plunge into a saucepan of boiling water for 1 minute, before draining and rinsing with cold water to stop the cooking process. Pat dry with a clean tea towel, then place in a large bowl with the air-dried noodles. Sprinkle with the soy sauce, mirin, sugar, sesame oil and the remaining curry powder. Toss until the noodles and beans are evenly coated.

- Now it's time to cook!

- In a wok, heat the rice bran oil over high heat until it's shimmering. Add the curried spring onion mix and stir constantly for 20 seconds. Add the mushroom mixture and stir-fry for another 2 minutes, or until the peas are bright green and no longer frozen.

- Toss the tofu or tofu-puffs through. Now add the noodles and cook for about 2 minutes, lifting and flipping the noodles so they heat through evenly.

- Pile into four warmed serving bowls. Sprinkle with the coriander, pop a lemon wedge on the side and serve immediately.

Provençal Potato Stew with Olives

SERVES 4

A simple and nourishing stew, rich with the flavours of southern France. Dish yourself up a big bowl and a glass of red wine, shut your eyes, and pretend you're on holiday with Léa Seydoux or Gaspard Ulliel ...

2 tablespoons olive oil, plus extra for drizzling

2 golden onions, sliced into thin half moons

2 celery stalks, cut into 1 cm chunks

4 garlic cloves, very thinly sliced

1 teaspoon dried oregano

3–4 thyme sprigs

8–10 waxy potatoes, such as Dutch cream, kipfler or nicola, peeled and cut into large chunks

½ cup red wine

1 tablespoon tomato paste

1 teaspoon brown sugar

2 large tomatoes, peeled and cut into large chunks

1 cup tomato passata

1½–2 cups vegan beef-style stock

4 bay leaves, fresh if possible

2 tablespoons vegan Worcestershire sauce

3–4 teaspoons sherry vinegar or red wine vinegar

1 cup kalamata olives, pitted

2 tablespoons capers, drained

½ bunch basil, roughly torn, reserving 4 sprigs to garnish

⅓ cup roughly chopped parsley

crusty bread, to serve

- In a heavy-based stockpot – cast iron if you have one! – heat the olive oil over medium heat. Add the onions and sauté for about 5 minutes, until they're mostly translucent. Add the celery and garlic and sauté for a further 1 minute. Stir in the oregano, then the thyme sprigs and potatoes, coating them with the olive oil.

- Turn the heat up to medium–high. When the pan is sizzling, tip in the red wine. Cook, stirring frequently, until the wine has mostly reduced; this should take about 4–5 minutes.

- Add the tomato paste and sugar, then stir for about 2 minutes, until they begin to caramelise slightly. Stir in the tomatoes, passata and 1½ cups of the stock, mixing well. Add the bay leaves and a few good grinds of black pepper, then bring to the boil.

- Immediately reduce the heat to a low simmer. Cover and cook for about 45 minutes, or up to 1 hour, until the potatoes are tender, but not falling apart. Stir occasionally to make sure the stew isn't sticking to the bottom of the pan; stir in the remaining stock if it looks a little dry.

- When the potatoes are tender, stir in the Worcestershire sauce, vinegar, olives, capers and basil and allow to warm through for about 5 minutes.

- Ladle into warmed serving bowls. Drizzle with a little good olive oil, sprinkle with the parsley and garnish with a basil sprig.

- Serve with fresh crusty bread to soak up all those tasty juices, and don't forget to warn diners about stray olive pits and bay leaves.

Variation

- For a potato and eggplant stew, cut one large eggplant into 1 cm dice and sauté in a frying pan in a tablespoon or two of olive oil until tender and golden brown. Mash half the eggplant with a fork, before pouring the whole lot into the stew when you add the passata and vegie stock. Proceed with the rest of the recipe as above.

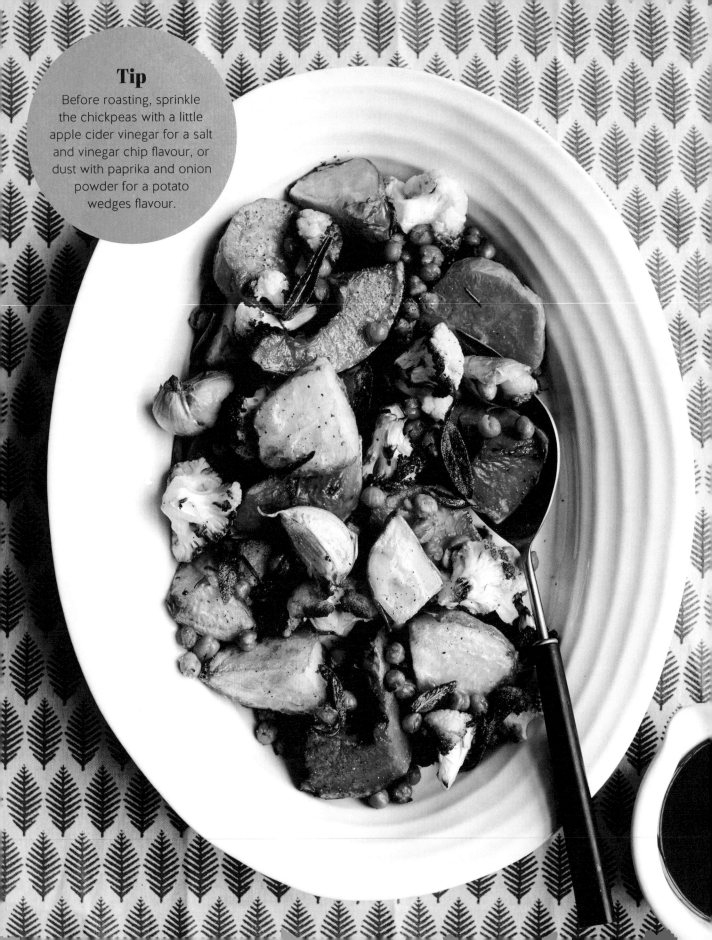

Tip

Before roasting, sprinkle the chickpeas with a little apple cider vinegar for a salt and vinegar chip flavour, or dust with paprika and onion powder for a potato wedges flavour.

Roast Vegetables with Garlic-herb Chickpeas

SERVES 2, OR 4 AS A SIDE

The trick to crispy roast vegies is to not overcrowd the baking dish, otherwise they'll steam and go soggy. Make sure there's plenty of space between them, and that the oven is nice and hot when you pop them in.

4 waxy potatoes, unpeeled
½ cauliflower, broken into small florets
1 large sweet potato
½ kent pumpkin
olive oil, for brushing
1 tablespoon dried rosemary
  or Italian herb mix
1 tablespoon vegan beef-style
  stock powder
6 garlic cloves, unpeeled and
  gently crushed
lemon wedges, to serve
Rich mushroom gravy (page 160),
  to serve

GARLIC-HERB CHICKPEAS

3–4 tablespoons olive oil
2 x 400 g tins chickpeas, rinsed
  and drained (see tip)
5–6 garlic cloves, unpeeled
a few fresh sage leaves

- Bring a saucepan of water to the boil. Scrub the potatoes clean, cut them into quarters and carefully drop them into the boiling water. Cook for about 10 minutes, or until a skewer pierces the potatoes easily, but they're not breaking apart.

- Meanwhile, steam the cauliflower for 3–5 minutes, or until just tender; you can do this by placing them in a steamer basket on top of the potatoes, or popping them in the microwave for about 1 minute.

- Preheat the oven to 220°C conventional, or 200°C fan-forced.

- Peel the sweet potato and pumpkin, cut into thick slices and spread over a large oiled baking tray with the blanched cauliflower, ensuring there is plenty of space between the vegies – you may even need to use two baking trays to prevent overcrowding.

- Drain the potatoes and use a fork to rough up the edges, so they get nice and crispy during cooking. Roll them in a little olive oil, sprinkle with the rosemary and stock powder, then place on the baking trays with the garlic cloves.

- Place the baking trays in the oven and bake for 40 minutes, or until the vegetables are a burnished golden brown.

- While the vegies are roasting, heat another baking tray in the oven, and prepare the chickpeas.

- Heat the olive oil in a heavy-based frying pan, then add the chickpeas. Cook, stirring occasionally, for a minute or two. Add the whole garlic cloves and stir constantly for 20–30 seconds, or until aromatic. Take the frying pan off the heat, add the sage leaves and stir to coat them in the oil.

- Once the vegies have been cooking for 20 minutes, pour the chickpea mixture onto the preheated baking tray and roast for the final 15–20 minutes of the vegie cooking time, or until the chickpeas turn golden. Stir them once or twice to stop them sticking.

- Remove the chickpeas from the oven, sprinkle with salt and pepper, then pour into a serving dish. Serve warm, with the roasted vegies, lemon wedges and lashings of hot gravy. The roasted garlic cloves will be creamy and mild – just pop them straight out of the skins for a sweet and savoury flavour hit!

Smoky Southern Black Beans with Coconut Rice

SERVES 4

So simple, and simply scrumptious. Beans and rice are staples of Latin American cuisine, and with good reason: they're hearty, warming, tasty and nutritious, packed full of protein and iron. This dish is very moreish on its own, or with a side salad; the smoky black beans are also fabulous in tacos and burritos.

1 red capsicum, seeded and
  membranes removed
1 onion, peeled
3 garlic cloves, peeled
¼ cup vegetable oil
1 teaspoon ground cumin
pinch of ground chilli, or to taste
1 bay leaf
2½ tablespoons vegetable stock
  powder
1½ tablespoons brown sugar
2 teaspoons liquid smoke
400 g tin diced tomatoes
2 x 400 g tins black beans (see tip),
  rinsed and drained
a handful of coriander, chopped

COCONUT RICE

2 cups jasmine or long-grain
  white rice
1 tablespoon sugar
2 cups coconut milk

- Finely dice the capsicum, onion and garlic, or roughly chop them, place in a blender and blitz for a few seconds until finely shredded.

- Heat the vegetable oil in a saucepan over medium heat. Pour in the capsicum mixture and simmer for a few minutes, until most of the excess liquid has reduced. Stir in the cumin, chilli and bay leaf and simmer for a minute longer.

- Add the stock powder, sugar and liquid smoke and mix until combined, then stir in the tomatoes and black beans. Simmer, uncovered, for 35 minutes, stirring occasionally.

- While the beans are simmering, prepare the coconut rice. Rinse the rice and place in a saucepan with the sugar and coconut milk. Add a pinch of salt, stir in 1 cup water and cook over low heat with the lid on for 20 minutes, or until the rice is soft.

- Turn off the heat and leave the rice to sit for a few minutes before serving.

- Garnish the smoky black beans with coriander and serve with the coconut rice.

Tip

This dish works well with other types of beans, such as pinto and kidney beans. Buying dried beans is a great way to save money and cut down on packaging. For advice on soaking dried beans, see page 61.

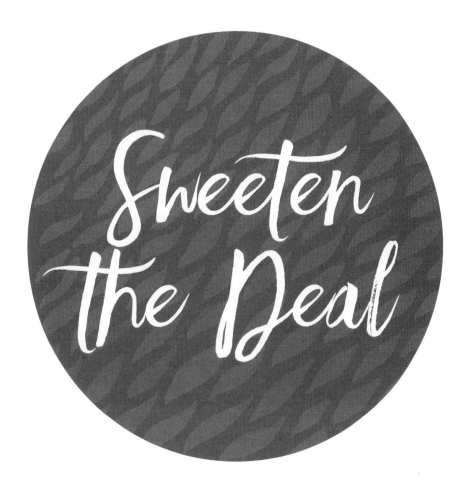

Sweeten the Deal

Light-as-air meringues. Syrup-sodden steamed puddings.
A show-stopping fudge cake. You've even got a healthy macadamia
cheesecake. It's never been easier to have your cake and eat it,
too, with these treats that are 100 per cent sweet to animals.

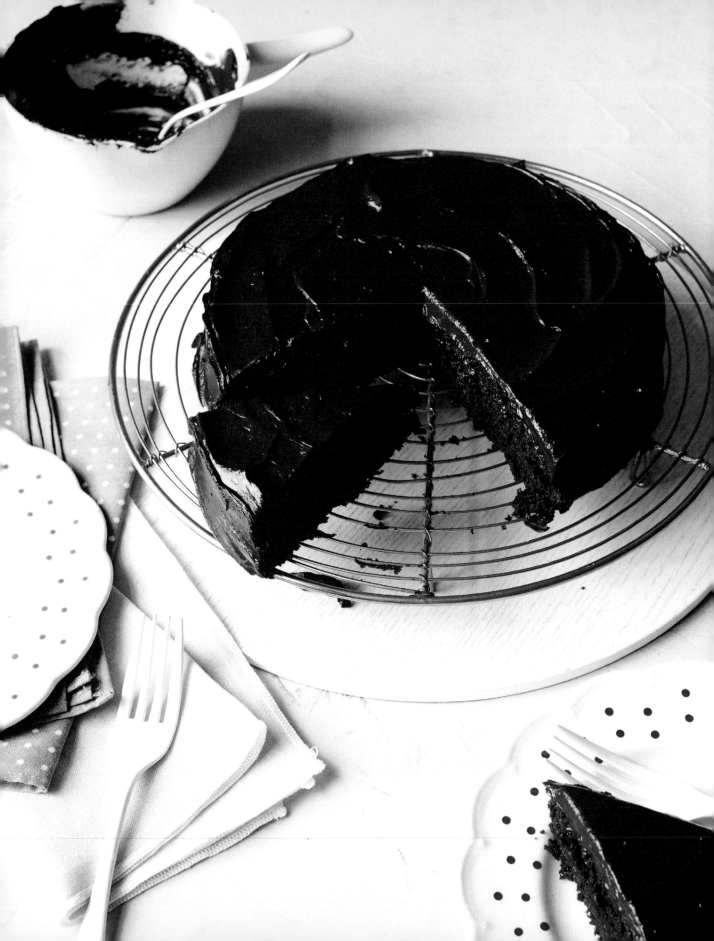

Chocolate Fudge Cake with Rich Ganache

SERVES 8

After a little indulgence? How does rich chocolate cake thickly frosted with the most delectable ganache sound? Perfect for a special occasion or naughty dessert with family at home, this cake requires few ingredients and is truly mouthwatering covered in a generous selection of berries and a light dusting of icing sugar. You can whip it up several hours ahead and pop the iced cake in the fridge to achieve an even more dense, moist texture.

1 cup plain flour
¼ cup cocoa powder
1 teaspoon bicarbonate of soda
1 teaspoon baking powder
½ teaspoon salt
1 cup sugar
⅓ cup rice bran oil
1 cup rice milk
fresh berries of your choice,
    to serve

COCONUT CREAM GANACHE
150 g dairy-free dark chocolate
    (at least 70% cocoa)
⅔ cup coconut cream

- Preheat the oven to 200°C conventional, or 180°C fan-forced. Carefully line a 20 cm round cake tin with baking paper. (This step is really important, because this cake has such a fudgy consistency and will otherwise stick to the pan.)

- Sift the flour, cocoa powder, bicarbonate of soda, baking powder and salt into a large bowl. Add the sugar and stir to combine.

- In a separate bowl, whisk together the rice bran oil and milk. Add the dry ingredients and gently fold them through until well combined.

- Pour the batter into the cake tin and bake for about 30 minutes, until the side of the cake has come away from the edge of the tin, the top isn't wobbly, and a skewer inserted in the centre comes out clean.

- Remove from the oven and leave until almost cooled, then turn the cake out of its tin and place on a serving plate.

- To make the coconut cream ganache, melt the chocolate by placing it in a heatproof bowl, set snugly over a saucepan of simmering water, but not touching the water, stirring until smooth. Meanwhile, in a separate small saucepan, gently heat the coconut cream. You don't want to boil it – just bring it up to a nice warm temperature, so it won't set the melted chocolate when you mix them together.

- Once the chocolate has melted, quickly whisk it into the warm coconut cream until well combined.

- Scrape the ganache out of the bowl, onto the cake, spreading it evenly all over. There is plenty of ganache, so it will be lovely and thick.

- Topping the cake with berries – try raspberries and strawberries! – is highly recommended to balance the rich sweetness of this lovely cake.

Tip
This cake will be much easier to slice if you make and ice it the day before, and refrigerate it overnight. Take it out of the fridge a few hours before serving so the ganache is nice and soft.

Recipe contributed by Melanie Baker, The Kind Cook

Caramel Slice

MAKES ABOUT 20 PIECES

Rich, gooey and intense, this isn't a slice for the faint of heart. One small sliver is enough – although you may find it hard to stop at one. The caramel layer can be made a day or two ahead and stored in the fridge.

GOLDEN CARAMEL

3 x 400 ml tins full-cream coconut
   milk or coconut cream
1 cup brown sugar
a pinch of sea salt
125 g coconut oil
⅓ cup golden syrup
2 teaspoons pure vanilla extract

COCONUT BISCUIT BASE

½ cup plain flour
¼ cup self-raising flour
½ cup cornflour
½ cup desiccated coconut
a pinch of sea salt
1 teaspoon pure vanilla extract
150 g coconut oil, melted

DARK CHOCOLATE TOPPING

200 g dairy-free dark chocolate
a pinch of sea salt
1 teaspoon vegetable or coconut oil

Tip

For a salted caramel slice, stir ½–1 teaspoon sea salt flakes through the cooled caramel before pouring on the base. Then, sprinkle an additional pinch or two of salt flakes over the slice before the chocolate sets.

- Preheat the oven to 200°C conventional, or 180°C fan-forced. Lightly grease a 24 cm square cake tin and line with baking paper.

- To make the golden caramel, shake the tins of coconut milk or cream, then pour the contents into a large saucepan. Stir in the sugar and salt. Bring to the boil over medium heat, stirring constantly, then reduce the heat to a gentle simmer. Leave to cook, stirring occasionally, until the coconut mixture has reduced by about half and thinly coats the back of the spoon. This could take up to 40 minutes, but you don't have to stir the whole time – just now and then to make sure the mixture isn't catching on the bottom of the pan.

- Once the mixture has thickened, stir in the coconut oil and golden syrup. Increase the heat to a high simmer and cook, stirring frequently, until the mixture thickens again. Remove from the heat and set aside to cool for a few minutes. Stir in the vanilla and cool to room temperature.

- To make the base, put the plain flour, self-raising flour and cornflour in a large mixing bowl and whisk to combine. Add the coconut and salt and whisk again. Mix the vanilla into the melted coconut oil, then pour over the dry ingredients. Stir until just combined – it should be fairly crumbly.

- Press the mixture into your cake tin, then bake for 10 minutes. Remove from the oven and allow to cool slightly.

- Holding a large spoon over the biscuit base, pour the caramel onto the spoon, letting it run onto the base. This helps distribute the caramel evenly, and stops you gouging a hole in the base. Bake for a further 15–17 minutes, or until the caramel is bubbling.

- Remove from the oven and set on a wire rack to cool. If the coconut oil in the caramel has separated out, don't panic – while it cools, just stir it gently to mix the caramel together again, taking care not to dredge up the biscuit base. Once cool, place the entire slice (still in its tin) in the fridge for a few hours, or overnight, to set the caramel layer.

- To make the chocolate topping, melt the chocolate in a microwave-safe bowl, or in a double-boiler, together with the salt and vegetable oil. Mix together, allow to cool slightly, then drizzle the chocolate over the caramel layer. Return to the fridge to set for at least 30 minutes.

- Remove the slice from the fridge at least 15 minutes before serving, so the chocolate doesn't crack when you try to cut it.

- This slice will keep for up to 5 days in the fridge in an airtight container.

Apple Rhubarb Crumble

SERVES 6

A crumble with extra crunch! Serve this one warm with dairy-free ice cream and everyone will be coming back for thirds. This basic recipe is your gateway to a world of fruit crumbles: leave out the rhubarb for a classic apple crumble, or add some berries, apricots, pears, peaches and/or sultanas to the baking dish before sprinkling the crumble mix on top. The almonds and coconut add flavour and texture to the topping, but you can always use extra oats instead.

4 apples, preferably Granny Smith; red apples will generally make the crumble sweeter
500 g rhubarb stalks
2 tablespoons sugar
1 teaspoon ground cinnamon

CRUMBLE TOPPING
¾ cup rolled oats
¾ cup plain flour
¾ cup shredded coconut
¾ cup flaked almonds
¾ cup white or raw sugar
1½ teaspoons ground cinnamon
a pinch of ground nutmeg
1 teaspoon pure vanilla extract
4 tablespoons dairy-free margarine

- Preheat the oven to 200°C conventional, or 180°C fan-forced.
- Peel and core the apples, then cut into wedges. Wash the rhubarb stalks and cut off any green tops. Cut the stalks into 3–5 cm lengths.
- Place the apple wedges in a saucepan. Sprinkle with the sugar and cinnamon and add enough water to cover the apples. Bring the water to a boil. As the water reaches boiling point, stir in the rhubarb. Reduce the heat to a simmer and cook for 3 minutes, or until the apple and rhubarb have softened.
- Pour off the liquid, then transfer the apples and rhubarb to a large baking dish, preferably one with deep sides.
- To prepare the crumble topping, combine the oats, flour, coconut, almonds, sugar and spices in a mixing bowl. Using your hands, mix in the vanilla and margarine, until the mixture clumps together, but still crumbles between your fingers.
- Sprinkle the crumble evenly over the apple mixture. Transfer to the oven and bake for 20–25 minutes, or until the crumble is golden.

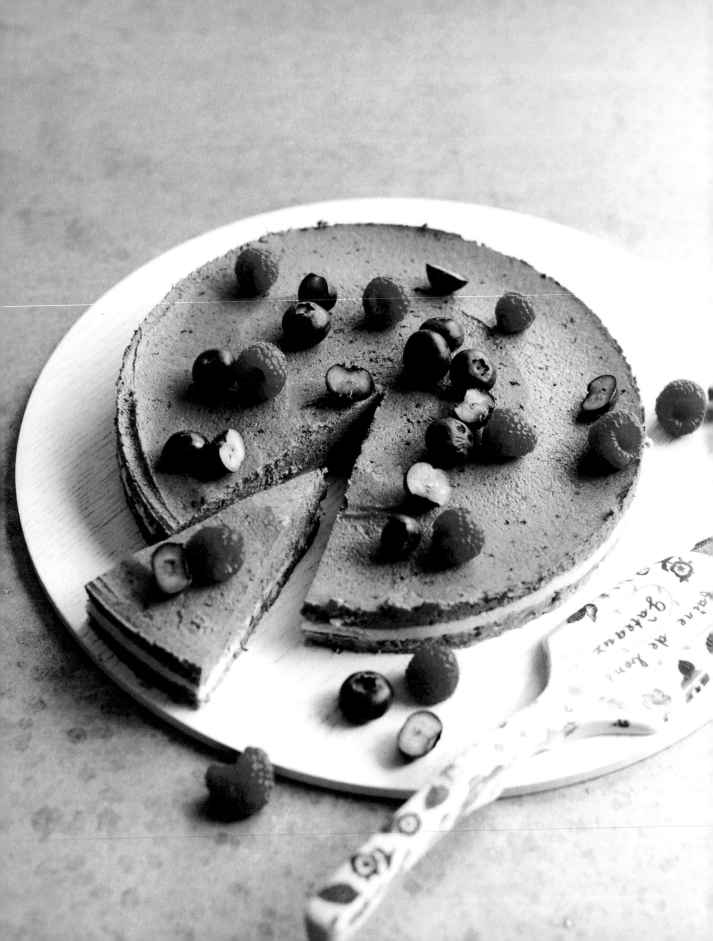

Raw Blueberry and Macadamia Cheesecake

MAKES ABOUT 10 SLICES

No oven? No worries! This decadent dessert is a deceptively easy win for those who aren't usually gifted in the baking department. Vibrantly hued blueberries create two distinctive colour layers, for a knockout presentation and flavour.

2 cups raw macadamias
½ cup maple syrup
juice of 1 lemon
¾ cup coconut oil, melted
1 teaspoon pure vanilla extract
1 cup fresh or frozen blueberries
fresh blueberries or raspberries,
   to garnish (optional)

NUTTY COCONUT BASE
1½ cups raw walnuts or almonds
5 dates, pitted
¼ cup desiccated coconut
1 tablespoon maple syrup

- Soak the macadamias in water for at least 2 hours, or preferably overnight.
- Grease a 20 cm spring-form cake tin with coconut oil.
- Put all the coconut base ingredients in a food processor and grind together until the mixture resembles a sticky crumble. Press the mixture firmly into the cake tin and set aside.
- Drain the macadamia nuts and place in a high-speed blender with the maple syrup, lemon juice, coconut oil and vanilla. Blend to a thick, creamy consistency, then pour half the macadamia mixture into the cake tin.
- Add the blueberries to the remaining mixture in the blender. Blend on high speed until the mixture is a vibrant purple colour and the blueberries have dissolved. Pour the mixture into the cake tin, smoothing and levelling the top with a spatula.
- Cover with plastic wrap and leave to set in the fridge for at least 2 hours. Decorate with extra blueberries or raspberries, if desired. Cut into slices to serve.
- This cheesecake will keep for a few days in the fridge.

Tip
Most berries work well in the cheesecake filling. Try strawberries or raspberries for a more subtle pink colour.

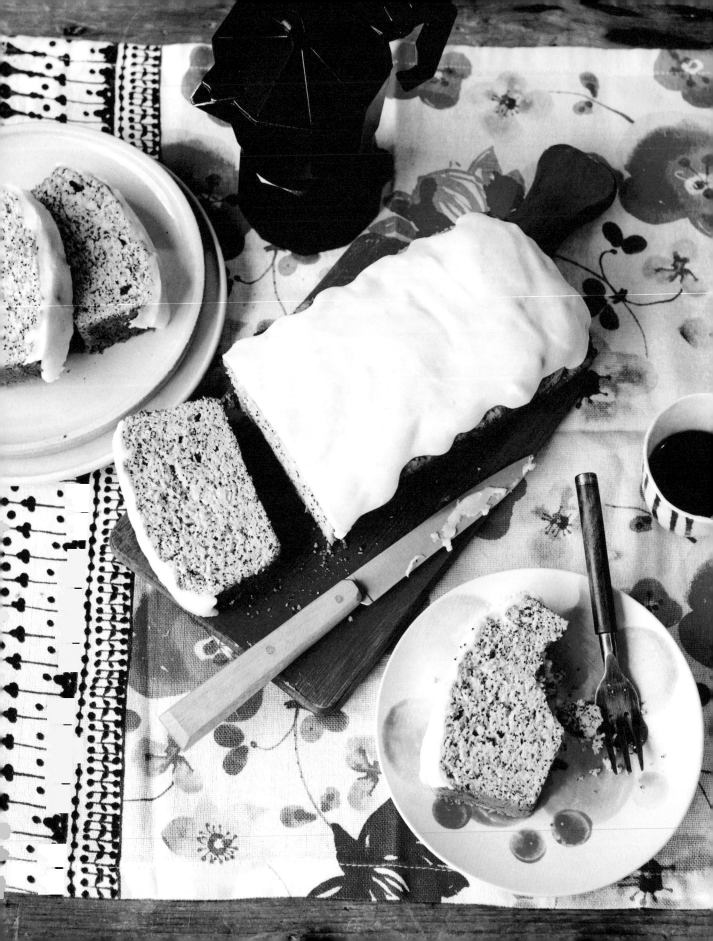

Lemon and Poppy Seed Cake

SERVES 10

How many times have you ordered poppy seed cake, only to find scant few seeds hiding in your slice? Never fear, a properly poppy-seeded cake is here, with this moist, citrusy cake, chock-full of poppy crunch. The lemon glaze is optional, but delicious.

2 cups plain flour
1 tablespoon baking powder
½ teaspoon bicarbonate of soda
¼ cup poppy seeds
¾ cup soy milk
zest and juice of 2 lemons
¾ cup coconut yoghurt
¾ cup brown sugar
2 teaspoons pure vanilla extract
4 tablespoons coconut oil, melted

LEMON GLAZE

½ teaspoon pure vanilla extract
1½ cups icing sugar, sifted
zest of 1 lemon
2 tablespoons lemon juice

- Preheat the oven to 180°C conventional, or 160°C fan-forced. Line a 22 cm loaf tin with baking paper.

- In a large bowl, sift together the flour, baking powder and bicarbonate of soda. Stir the poppy seeds through.

- In another bowl, whisk together the soy milk, lemon zest and lemon juice, coconut yoghurt, sugar and vanilla until the sugar has dissolved. Whisk in the melted coconut oil until combined. Pour the mixture into the dry ingredients and stir until just combined, taking care not to overmix.

- Pour the batter into the loaf tin and bake for about 40 minutes, or until a skewer inserted into the centre comes out clean.

- Remove from the oven and allow to cool completely in the tin, before turning out.

- To make the lemon glaze, beat the vanilla, sifted icing sugar and lemon zest together. Slowly add the lemon juice until the mixture is smooth and the desired consistency is reached.

- Drizzle the lemon glaze over the cooled cake. Cut into slices to serve.

- This cake will keep for 1–2 days in an airtight container.

Tip

For an even easier lemon glaze, simply mix sifted icing sugar with lemon juice until smooth.

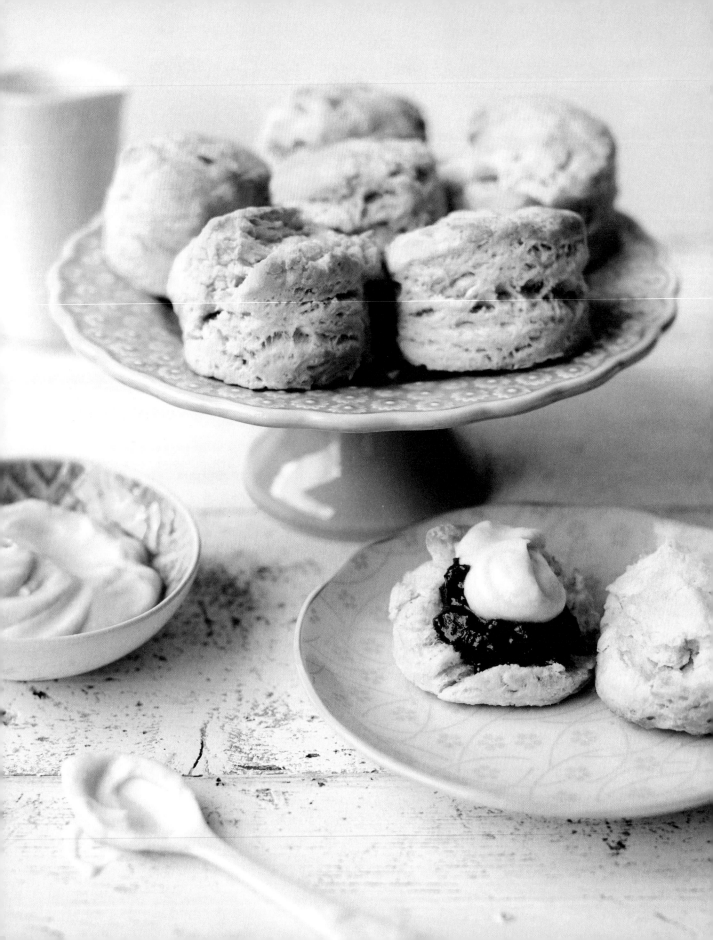

Scones with Jam and Vanilla Coconut Cream

MAKES 10–12 SCONES

Guests arriving in half an hour, all you have in the cupboard is a packet of stale biscuits and there's not enough time to make a cake – what do you do? Make scones! From go to whoa you can have these on the table, piping hot and ready to be devoured, in less than 30 minutes. Spread with your favourite jam, pile high with cow-friendly coconut cream and watch as everyone reaches for another.

2 cups self-raising flour
3 tablespoons solid coconut oil
1 cup soy milk, plus extra for brushing
your favourite jam, to serve
Whipped vanilla coconut cream
    (from the Meringue nests recipe
    on page 240), to serve

- Preheat the oven to 240°C conventional, or 220°C fan-forced. Line a three-sided scone tray with baking paper. (At a pinch, you can also use a very shallow four-sided tray.)

- Sift the flour and a pinch of salt into a large bowl. Using your fingertips, rub the solid coconut oil into the flour mixture. You're aiming for a rough breadcrumb texture here, but you don't have to be too exact about this – it's better to underwork than overwork the mixture.

- Make a little well in the centre and pour in the milk. Gently stir with a knife until the mixture is just barely combined, then turn out onto a floured surface. Gently press the mixture until it just holds together, then pat into a circle about 2 cm thick. With a 5 cm round biscuit cutter (or a glass!), cut out your scones, pressing the leftover dough scraps together gently until you've used up as much of the dough as you can. You should have enough dough for 10–12 scones.

- Place the scones, just touching each other, on your baking tray. Brush the tops with an extra tablespoon or so of milk, then pop them in the oven and bake for 10–15 minutes. They say a watched pot never boils – but unwatched scones always burn, so perch like a hawk and watch through the oven door until your scones have risen and are a beautiful burnished gold on top.

- Remove from the oven, split in half, then slather with the jam and coconut cream.

Tip

For delicious date scones, replace half the flour with wholemeal self-raising flour, add ½ teaspoon ground cinnamon, then mix through 1 cup chopped pitted dates after you've rubbed in the coconut oil.

Sticky Date Pudding

SERVES 8

From pub counter meals to Sunday family lunches, date pudding is a classic Aussie favourite. Sweet, sticky and ever-so-slightly spiced, this steamed pud is delicious on its own, or with a big scoop of ice cream and a hearty drizzle of caramel sauce. And the best bit? Leftovers – if there are any – are perfect for a cheeky breakfast …

1½ cups dates, pitted and chopped into small pieces
1 teaspoon bicarbonate of soda
100 g dairy-free margarine
50 g brown sugar
1 teaspoon pure vanilla extract
200 g self-raising flour
1 teaspoon ground ginger
½ teaspoon ground cinnamon
½ teaspoon ground nutmeg

CARAMEL SAUCE

¼ teaspoon pure vanilla extract
400 g tin condensed coconut milk
   (available from most supermarkets)
¼ cup brown sugar
¼ teaspoon salt

- Preheat the oven to 200°C conventional, or 180°C fan-forced.
- Bring 1½ cups water to the boil in a saucepan. Add the dates and simmer for 2–3 minutes. Stir in the bicarbonate of soda, remove from the heat and leave to sit for 15 minutes.
- In a bowl, cream the margarine and sugar together, either by hand with a wooden spoon, or using an electric mixer, taking care not to overmix. Add the vanilla and the date mixture, then fold the flour and spices through.
- Pour the mixture into an 18 cm square baking dish.
- Fill a large roasting tin two-thirds full with hot water, then place the baking dish inside it. Completely cover the whole thing with foil, to create a steam bath to ensure the pudding stays lovely and moist in the oven.
- Carefully transfer to the oven and bake for about 1 hour, or until a skewer inserted in the centre of the pudding comes out clean. Be careful when testing the pudding as the water will be very hot and the roasting tin heavy.
- Near serving time, place all the caramel sauce ingredients in a saucepan. Bring to a simmer over medium heat and cook, stirring, for 5–10 minutes, until thickened.
- Scoop the warm pudding into serving bowls, using a large spoon. Serve with the caramel sauce, and dairy-free ice cream if desired.

Peanut Butter Choc-chip Ice Cream

SERVES 2

No wonder this sweet treat is often called 'nice cream'! Using frozen bananas as the base, it's a simple and refreshing summer dessert that's creamy and indulgent.

3 ripe bananas, chopped and frozen
(see tip)
1½ tablespoons crunchy peanut butter
3–4 tablespoons soy milk
2 tablespoons dairy-free dark
choc chips

- Put the bananas, peanut butter and 3 tablespoons of the soy milk in a high-speed blender.

- Blend on low speed for 2–3 minutes, until the mixture becomes creamy, with a soft-serve texture. Add the remaining tablespoon of soy milk only if needed to keep the mixture moving – you don't want it too liquidy. You may need to occasionally stop blending, and use a spatula to push the mixture onto the blade to ensure it blends evenly.

- Use a spatula to scrape the mixture into a mixing bowl. Stir the choc chips through.

- Serve immediately, or for a firmer ice cream, freeze for at least 1 hour in an airtight freezer-safe container, and remove from the freezer 5–10 minutes before serving.

Variations

- For raspberry mint ice cream, use 1½ frozen bananas, 1 cup frozen raspberries, 3 tablespoons soy milk and a few fresh mint leaves; add rice malt syrup, sugar or agave syrup to taste.

- For cinnamon vanilla ice cream, use 3 frozen bananas, 3 tablespoons soy milk, 1 teaspoon pure vanilla extract and ½ teaspoon ground cinnamon; add maple syrup to taste, if desired.

- Invent your own flavour using nut butters, cocoa or cacao, fresh or dried fruit, fresh herbs or spices; you might need a little extra soy milk for dry additions. Play with toppings such as shredded coconut, chopped nuts or cacao nibs.

Tip

When bananas are abundant, very ripe ones can be peeled, chopped and frozen in zip-lock bags, ready to use in smoothies and recipes such as this.

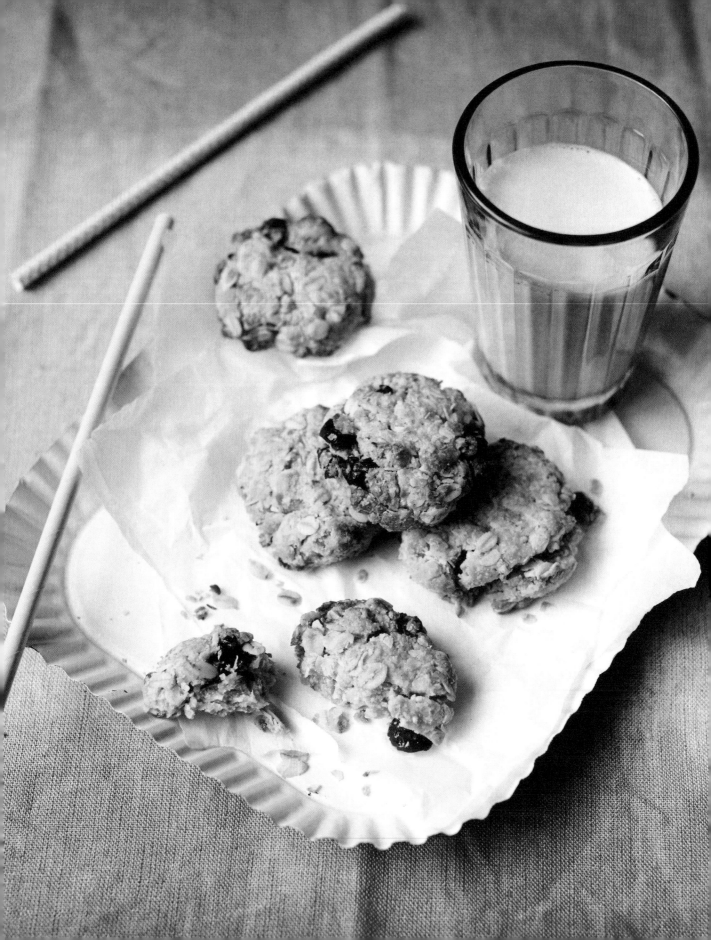

Cranberry, Apricot and Rolled Oat Cookies

MAKES 20

You can use any dried fruit in these wonderfully versatile cookies; add some dark chocolate chips for a sweeter snack, or trade white flour for the wholemeal if you prefer. These ones keep well for up to a week and are terrific in lunchboxes.

1 cup wholemeal self-raising flour

1 cup rolled oats

1 tablespoon brown sugar

½ cup desiccated coconut

½ cup finely chopped dried cranberries

½ cup finely chopped dried apricots

120 g dairy-free margarine

⅓ cup golden syrup

1 teaspoon pure vanilla extract

- Preheat the oven to 190°C conventional, or 170°C fan-forced. Line a large baking tray with baking paper.

- In a large bowl, mix together the flour, oats, sugar, coconut and dried fruits. Set aside.

- Melt the margarine in a microwave-safe bowl, or in a saucepan over low heat. Stir in the golden syrup and vanilla until well combined, then pour over the flour mixture and stir until combined.

- Roll teaspoons of the mixture into balls and place on the baking tray. Flatten slightly with a fork, then bake for 10–12 minutes, or until lightly golden. Take care not to overcook the biscuits, or they'll be crunchy, rather than chewy.

- Remove from the oven and leave to cool on a wire rack, before storing in an airtight container. The biscuits will be soft when they come out of the oven, but will harden on cooling.

Meringue Nests with Whipped Coconut Cream and Fresh Fruits

MAKES 12

Light as air and sweet as a kiss, these meringues have been given a contemporary, compassionate twist; you'll never guess their secret ingredient! Filled with pillow-soft whipped coconut cream, and adorned with fresh seasonal fruits, they make an elegant end to a dinner party, or a welcome appearance at lazy summer barbecues.

the 'aquafaba' (liquid) from a 400 g tin of chickpeas, drained and strained
150 g icing sugar
150 g golden caster sugar (or regular caster sugar)
1 teaspoon cream of tartar
1 teaspoon pure vanilla extract
fresh berries and cherries, to serve (see tip)

WHIPPED VANILLA COCONUT CREAM

250 ml coconut cream, refrigerated in the tin
1 teaspoon pure vanilla extract
maple syrup (optional)

- Preheat the oven to 120°C conventional, or 100°C fan-forced. Line two baking trays with baking paper.

- Put the aquafaba in an extremely clean large bowl. Using electric beaters, beat on high speed for about 5 minutes, or until soft peaks form.

- While continuing to beat, gradually add the icing sugar, then the caster sugar. You may not need all the sugar – stop if the mixture is getting too thick.

- Once the sugar is incorporated and has dissolved, sprinkle in the cream of tartar and the vanilla. Continue to beat until stiff peaks form.

- Scoop the meringue mixture into a piping bag. You may need to do this in two batches.

- Pipe nests of meringue onto the lined baking trays. To do this, pipe a 'base' of concentric circles to about 10 cm wide, then pipe around the outside edge, about three spirals high, to create a 'nest' shape.

- Bake for about 2 hours, depending on the size of your nests, keeping an eye on them to make sure they don't start to brown. Switch the oven off, but leave the meringues in there, with the door open a little, for a further 30 minutes. They should be light and dry when you remove them from the oven.

- The meringues can be made a day or two ahead and stored in an airtight container until required.

- Just before assembling your meringue nests, make the whipped vanilla coconut cream. Put the coconut cream and vanilla in a bowl and, using electric beaters, whisk on high speed until thickened. If using the maple syrup, add it teaspoon by teaspoon, until the desired level of sweetness is achieved; keep in mind that the meringues themselves are very sweet.

- Spoon the whipped vanilla coconut cream into the meringue nests, top with your choice of fresh fruits and serve.

Tip

Vary the fruit toppings to suit the season. For a classic Aussie pav, top with fresh mango, kiwifruit slices and a drizzle of passionfruit pulp.

Avocado, Lime and Cashew Slice

SERVES 8

Imagine yourself on a tropical island holiday, lying on the beach eating dates ... with a big, icy glass garnished with a lime wedge in your hand ... having coconut oil rubbed into your shoulders by a golden god and ... okay, pause right there. Now imagine that holiday condensed into a slice. This is that slice. Smooth and creamy, with a sucker punch of zesty lime to keep things interesting. Serve it up and see if anyone can guess the mystery ingredient – no hints!

1 avocado

1 cup cashews, soaked in hot water for 15 minutes, then drained

2 tablespoons grated lime zest

¼ cup lime juice

100 ml agave syrup

¼ teaspoon sea salt

2 teaspoons pure vanilla extract

3 tablespoons coconut oil, melted

a handful of finely shredded dried coconut, for sprinkling

ALMOND CRUST

1 cup finely shredded dried coconut

1 cup almond meal

6 pitted medjool dates

¼ teaspoon sea salt

2 tablespoons lemon zest

¼ cup lemon juice

1 teaspoon pure vanilla extract

- Preheat the oven to 180°C conventional, or 160°C fan-forced. Line a 28 cm x 18 cm slice tin with baking paper.

- Place all the almond crust ingredients in a food processor and blend until the mixture starts to hold together. Press the base evenly into the slice tin and set aside.

- Clean out the food processor. Add the flesh from the avocado, along with the cashews, lime zest, lime juice, agave syrup, salt and vanilla. Blend until smooth, then slowly add the coconut oil and process for a further minute.

- Spoon the filling into the slice tin, spreading it all over the base. It doesn't have to be perfectly flat – it's nice if it's a little messy, as the peaks will go golden brown in the oven.

- Bake for 15–20 minutes, or until the filling is lightly golden brown. Remove from the oven and leave to cool completely before taking it out of the tin.

- Sprinkle the dried coconut over the slice. Cut into portions and serve warm, or chill the slice in the fridge, where it will set firmly.

- This slice will keep for up to 3 days in an airtight container in the fridge; leave to soften at room temperature for 15 minutes before eating.

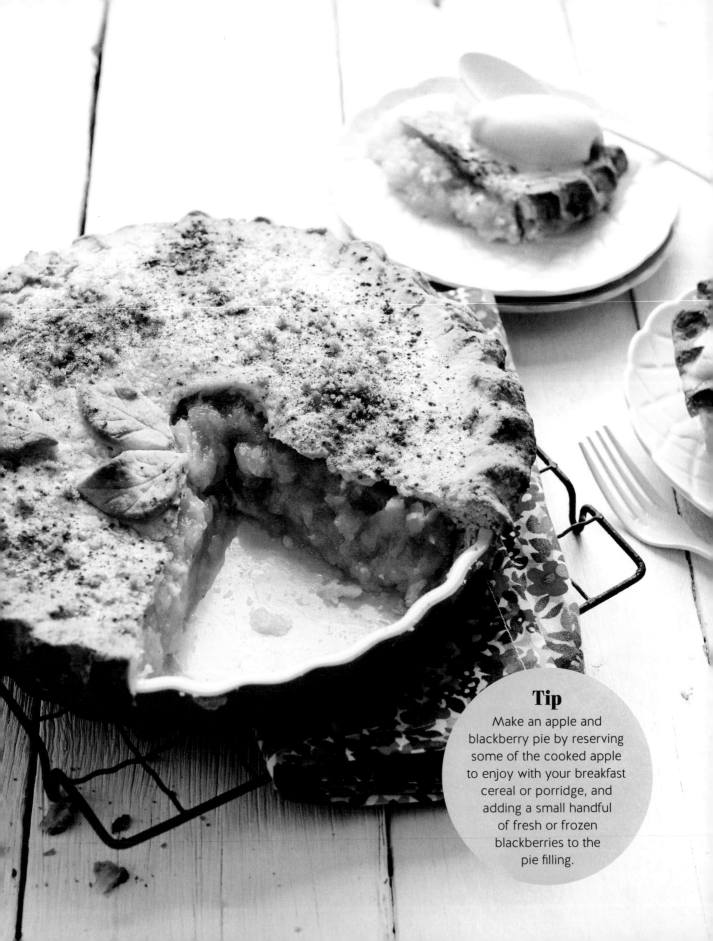

Tip

Make an apple and blackberry pie by reserving some of the cooked apple to enjoy with your breakfast cereal or porridge, and adding a small handful of fresh or frozen blackberries to the pie filling.

Golden-crusted Apple Pie

SERVES 6-8

A pure and simple old-fashioned pie, with a crispy golden crust. It is delicious
on its own, or served with a scoop of dairy-free vanilla ice cream.

2 kg Granny Smith apples, or other
   in-season cooking apples
½ cup brown sugar

GOLDEN-CRUST PASTRY

⅔ cup coconut oil, softened
   but not melted
½ cup brown sugar
1 teaspoon pure vanilla extract
1 cup plain flour, plus extra for dusting
1 cup self-raising flour
1¼ tablespoons cornflour
½ cup oat milk
¾–1 teaspoon ground cinnamon,
   for sprinkling
1 tablespoon raw sugar, for sprinkling

- Preheat the oven to 200°C conventional, or 180°C fan-forced. Grease a 25 cm pie dish.

- Peel the apples and cut into odd-shaped slices; the aim is for some of the apples to break down into a sauce, and other pieces to retain more body for texture.

- Place the apple pieces in a large saucepan with a scant ¼–⅓ cup water. Cover and cook over medium-high heat for about 20 minutes, stirring frequently to stop the apples sticking to the pan and to ensure they cook evenly. When the apples are tender, add the sugar and stir until dissolved. Set aside while preparing the pastry.

- In a bowl, beat the softened coconut oil and brown sugar using a hand beater or electric mixer until creamy. Add the vanilla and mix well.

- Sift together the plain flour, self-raising flour and cornflour. Alternating with the oat milk, add the sifted flour mixture to the beaten coconut oil mixture, mixing well after each addition, until all the flour and oat milk have been added.

- On a generously floured work surface, roll the pastry out to about 1–1.5 cm thick. Cut off and set aside one-quarter of the pastry for the pie lid.

- Use the remaining pastry to line the greased pie dish, making sure it overlaps the edge slightly, so you can attach the lid. Fill with the warm apple mixture, then pat the reserved pastry into a round lid shape and place on top; don't worry if it breaks, just pinch it back together. This is meant to be a rustic pie, after all! Use a fork or your fingers to press the top and bottom pastry edges together. Using a sharp knife or a fork, poke a few holes in the pie lid to let the steam out.

- Sprinkle the cinnamon over the pastry, then the raw sugar. Place in the oven and bake for 40–45 minutes, rotating the pie to ensure even cooking, and loosely covering the top with foil if it starts getting too brown.

- Remove from the oven. Leave to cool for a few minutes before serving.

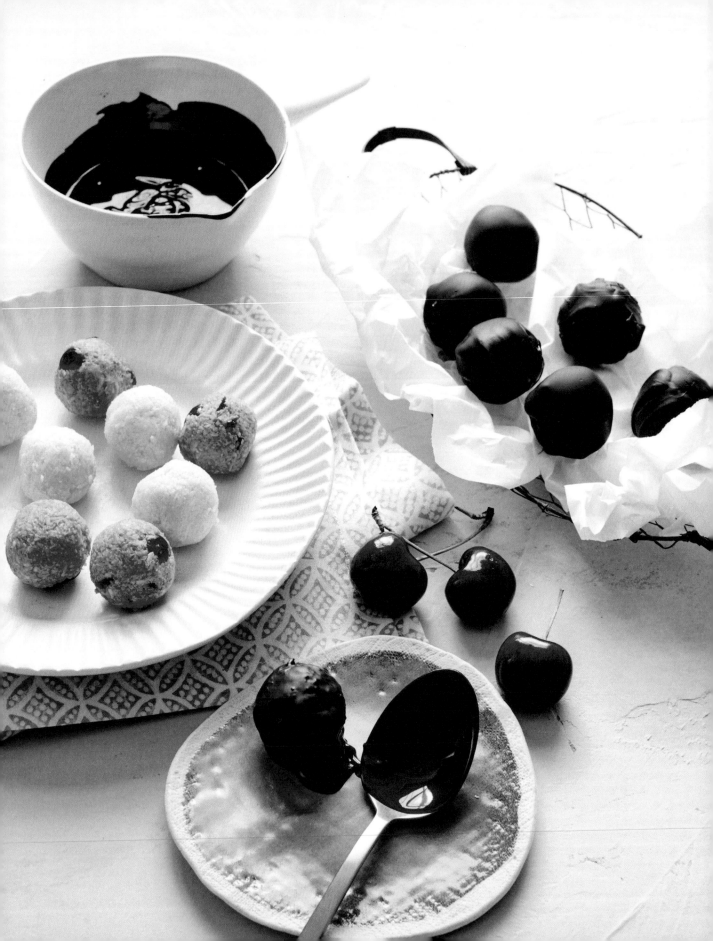

Coconut and Cherry Nice Truffles

MAKES ABOUT 16 TRUFFLES

*Rich, smooth chocolate encloses a creamy, vanilla-scented coconut filling for
a tiny taste of heaven. For an extra-special grown-up treat, soak the glacé cherries
in brandy before adding to the coconut mix. Just try stopping at one.*

2 cups shredded coconut
2 teaspoons pure vanilla extract
¼ teaspoon salt
4 tablespoons coconut oil, melted
3 tablespoons agave syrup
2 tablespoons full-cream
  coconut milk
75 g glacé cherries, roughly chopped
a drop of red food colouring
  (optional)
300 g dairy-free dark chocolate

● Line a large baking tray with baking paper.

● Put the coconut, vanilla and salt in a blender. Pour in the coconut oil, agave syrup and coconut milk, then pulse in 1-second bursts until the mixture is very roughly combined. You're not aiming for a smooth paste here; it's important to keep some coconut texture. Don't worry if there are a few dry patches.

● Using a spatula, scoop the mixture out of the blender, into a mixing bowl. Get your hands in there and give it all a good squish to make sure the vanilla, coconut milk and oil are evenly distributed. Divide the mixture into two even portions. To one portion, add the cherries and red food colouring, if using.

● Now, the fun bit! Roll the mixtures into teaspoon-sized balls and place on the baking tray; a pretty touch with the cherry mixture is to shape it into love hearts by firmly pressing a spoonful into a small heart-shaped biscuit cutter and gently easing them onto the baking tray. Pop the tray in the fridge for at least 30 minutes to allow the coconut filling to set.

● Once the coconut centres are cold, melt the chocolate, either in the microwave or in a double-boiler on your stovetop, then remove from the heat.

● Working fairly quickly before the chocolate sets, drop one coconut ball into the chocolate and roll to cover. Scoop it out with a fork and allow any excess chocolate to drip off before placing it back on the baking tray.

● Once you've choc-dipped all your truffles, place the tray back in the fridge to set the chocolate. You won't have to wait long – they'll be ready to devour in T-minus 5 minutes and counting.

Super Easy Strawberry Cheesecake

SERVES 8

Here's proof that delicious desserts don't need to be difficult: this baked dairy-free cheesecake requires only five ingredients and is a perfect mix of sweet, creamy and tart. It's versatile too – simply swap the strawberry jam for any variety that takes your fancy. Add extra flair by topping with fresh fruit, or even a thin layer of jam for extra sweetness.

250 g biscuits (such as digestive biscuits), crushed
100 g dairy-free margarine, melted
600–700 g dairy-free cream cheese
4 tablespoons strawberry jam
1 tablespoon cornflour

- Preheat the oven to 180°C conventional, or 160°C fan-forced. Line a 22 cm baking dish or spring-form cake tin with baking paper.

- Mix the crushed biscuits and melted margarine together in a bowl. Press the mixture into the baking dish, to create an even base.

- Place the remaining ingredients in a bowl and mix together well. Spoon the mixture into the baking dish.

- Transfer to the oven and bake for 25 minutes, or until the filling is set.

- Remove from the oven and set aside to cool, then set in the fridge for at least 2 hours, or overnight. Cut into slices to serve.

- This cheesecake will keep for several days in the fridge.

Notes

1   ABC Rural | NSW Country Hour, (2015) *Demand for meat alternatives and soy products growing in Australia.* [online] Available at: www.abc.net.au/news/2015-08-31/meat-alternatives/6726756 [Accessed 25 Sept 2016]

2   Sydney Morning Herald | Consumer Affairs, (2016). *Australia is the third-fastest growing vegan market in the world.* [online] Available at: www.smh.com.au/business/consumer-affairs/australia-is-the-thirdfastest-growing-vegan-market-in-the-world-20160601-gp972u.html [Accessed 25 Sept 2016]

3   Mirror | Diet, (2016). *A quarter of the nation will be vegetarian within 25 years, research claims.* [online] Available at: www.mirror.co.uk/news/uk-news/quarter-nation-vegetarian-within-25-7977430 [Accessed 25 Sept 2016]

4   Obesity Australia, (2016). *Adult obesity in Australia.* [online] Available at: www.obesityaustralia.org/LiteratureRetrieve.aspx?ID=199407 [Accessed 17 Aug 2016].

5   Better Health Channel and The Royal Children's Hospital Melbourne, (2014). *Obesity in children – causes.* [online] Available at: www.betterhealth.vic.gov.au/health/healthyliving/obesity-in-children-causes [Accessed 16 Aug 2016].

6   Pi-Sunyer (MD), X. (2009). The medical risks of obesity. *Postgraduate Medicine,* [online] Volume 121 (6), 21–33. Available at: www.ncbi.nlm.nih.gov/pmc/articles/PMC2879283/ [Accessed 17 Aug 2016]

7   Berkow, S.E and Barnard, N. (2006). Vegetarian diets and weight status. *Nutrition Reviews,* [online] Volume 64 (4), 175-88. Available at: www.ncbi.nlm.nih.gov/pubmed/16673753. Referenced at: www.ncbi.nlm.nih.gov/pmc/articles/PMC3048091/#b28-cmr-3-001. [Accessed 12 Aug 2016].

8   Australian Institute of Health and Welfare, (2016). *Leading causes of death.* [online] Available at: www.aihw.gov.au/deaths/leading-causes-of-death/. [Accessed 16 Aug 2016].

9   Crowe F.L, Appleby P.N, Travis R.C and Key T.J. (2013). Risk of hospitalization or death from ischemic heart disease among British vegetarians and nonvegetarians: results from the EPIC-Oxford cohort study. *American Journal of Clinical Nutrition,* [online] Volume 97 (3), 597-603. Available at: www.ncbi.nlm.nih.gov/pubmed/23364007 [Accessed 12 Aug 2016].

10 Diabetes Australia, (2015). *Diabetes in Australia.* [online] Available at: www.diabetesaustralia.com.au/diabetes-in-australia [Accessed 16 Aug 2016].

11 Tripp, C., Levin, S. (2012) Preparing to prescribe plant-based diets for diabetes prevention and treatment. *Diabetes Spectrum,* [online]. Volume 25 (1), 38-44. Available at: spectrum.diabetesjournals.org/content/25/1/38 [Accessed 25 Sept 2016]

12 Cancer Council Australia, (2016). *Facts and figures: Cancer in Australia.* [online] Available at: www.cancer.org.au/about-cancer/what-is-cancer/facts-and-figures.html [Accessed 16 Aug 2016].

13 Anand, P., Kunnumakara, A., Sundaram, C., Harikumar, K., Tharakan, S., Lai, O., Sung, B., and Aggarwal, B. (2008). Cancer is a preventable disease that requires major lifestyle changes. *Pharmaceutical research,* [online]. Volume 25 (9), 2097-2116. Available at: www.ncbi.nlm.nih.gov/pmc/articles/PMC2515569/ [Accessed 17 Aug 2016]

14 The Age | Epicure, (2008). *Tantalising flavours override taste of fear.* [online] Available at: www.theage.com.au/news/epicure/tantalising-flavours-override-taste-of-fear/2008/08/09/1218139176701.html [Accessed 17 Aug 2016]

15 World Health Organization | International Agency for Research on Cancer, (2015). *IARC Monographs evaluate consumption of red meat and processed meat.* Available at: www.iarc.fr/en/media-centre/pr/2015/pdfs/pr240_E.pdf [Accessed on 12 Aug 2016]

16 World Health Organization (WHO), The Food and Agricultural Organization (FAO) and World Organisation for Animal Health (OIE) (2003). *Joint FAO/OIE/WHO expert workshop on non-human antimicrobial usage and antimicrobial resistance: Scientific assessment.* [online] Available at: www.oie.int/doc/en_document.php?numrec=1046703 [Accessed 16 Aug 2016]

17 Australian Pesticides and Veterinary Medicines Authority, (2014). *Quantity of antimicrobial products sold for veterinary use in Australia.* [online] Available at: archive.apvma.gov.au/publications/reports/docs/antimicrobial_sales_report_march-2014.pdf [Accessed 4 Oct 2016]

18 Lymbery, P. and Oakeshott, I. (2014). *Farmageddon: The true cost of cheap meat.* New York: Bloomsbury, p. 139.

19 World Health Organization (WHO), The Food and Agricultural Organization (FAO) and World Animal Health Organisation (OIE) (2003). *Joint FAO/OIE/WHO expert workshop on non-human antimicrobial usage and antimicrobial resistance: Scientific assessment.* [online] Available at: www.oie.int/doc/en_document.php?numrec=1046703 [Accessed 16 Aug 2016]

20 World Health Organization, (2011). *Campylobacter.* [online] Available at: www.who.int/mediacentre/factsheets/fs255/en/ [Accessed 16 Aug 2016]

21 Food Standards Australia New Zealand (FSANZ) and South Australian Research and Development Institute, (2010). *Baseline survey on the prevalence and concentration of Salmonella and Campylobacter in chicken meat on-farm and at primary processing.* [online] Available at: www.foodstandards.gov.au/publications/documents/Poultry%20survey%20rept%20March%202010.pdf [Accessed 16 Aug 2016]

22 Australian Government | Department of Health, (2010). *8 Food poisoning and contamination.* [online] Available at: www.health.gov.au/internet/publications/publishing.nsf/Content/ohp-enhealth-manual-atsi-cnt-l~ohp-enhealth-manual-atsi-cnt-l-ch3~ohp-enhealth-manual-atsi-cnt-l-ch3.8 [Accessed 16 Aug 2016]

23 Pimentel, D. and Pimentel, M. (2003). Sustainability of meat-based and plant-based diets and the environment. *The American Journal of Clinical Nutrition,* [online] 78 (suppl), 660S-3S. Available at: ajcn.nutrition.org/content/78/3/660S.full.pdf [Accessed 21 Aug 2016].

24 Food and Agriculture Organization of the United Nations (FAO), (2006). *Livestock's long shadow: Environmental issues and options.* [online] Available at: www.fao.org/docrep/010/a0701e/a0701e00.HTM [Accessed 19 Aug 2016]

25 Desai, M., Rogers, J., and Smith, K. (2015). Applications of a joint CO2 and CH4 climate debt metric: Insights into global patterns and mitigation priorities. *Global Environmental Change,* [online] Volume 35, 176-189. Available at: ehsdiv.sph.berkeley.edu/krsmith/publications/2015/Desai%20_climate_debt_metric.pdf [Accessed 20 Aug 2016].

26 Food and Agriculture Organization of the United Nations (FAO), (2006). *Livestock's long shadow: Environmental issues and options.* [online] Available at: www.fao.org/

docrep/010/a0701e/a0701e00.HTM [Accessed 19 Aug 2016].

27 Shindell, D., Faluvegi, G., Koch, D., Schmidt, G., Unger, N., and Bauer, S. (2009). Improved attribution of climate forcing to emissions. *Science*, [online] Volume 326 (5953), 716-18. Available at: science.sciencemag.org/content/326/5953/716.full [Accessed 18 Aug 2016].

28 Wellesley, L., Froggatt, A., and Happer, C. (2015). *Changing climate, changing diets: Pathways to lower meat consumption.* [online] Available at: www.chathamhouse.org/publication/changing-climate-changing-diets [Accessed 18 Aug 2016].

29 Waite, R. (2016). *How I tweaked my diet to cut its environmental footprint in half.* [online]. World Resources Institute. Available at: www.wri.org/blog/2016/04/how-i-tweaked-my-diet-cut-its-environmental-footprint-half [Accessed 18 Aug 2016].

30 Pew Commission on Industrial Farm Animal Production (PCIFAP), (2008). *Putting meat on the table: Industrial farm animal production in America.* [online] Available at: www.pewtrusts.org/~/media/legacy/uploadedfiles/peg/publications/report/pcifapfinalpdf.pdf [Accessed 18 Aug 2016].

31 Pew Commission on Industrial Farm Animal Production (PCIFAP), (2008). *Putting meat on the table: Industrial farm animal production in America.* [online] Available at: www.pewtrusts.org/~/media/legacy/uploadedfiles/peg/publications/report/pcifapfinalpdf.pdf [Accessed 18 Aug 2016].

32 Rosegrant, M., Ximing Cai, S. and Cline, S. (2002). *Global water outlook to 2025: Averting an impending crisis.* [online] Available at: ageconsearch.umn.edu/bitstream/16144/1/fp02ro01.pdf [Accessed 19 Aug 2016].

33 Herrero, M., Wirsenius, S., Henderson, B., Rigolot, C., Thornton, P., Havlík, P., de Boer, I., and Gerber, P. (2015). Livestock and the environment: What have we learned in the past decade? *Annual Review of Environment and Resources*, [online] Volume 40, 177-202. Available at: www.annualreviews.org/doi/full/10.1146/annurev-environ-031113-093503 [Accessed 18 Aug 2016].

34 (Calculations based on average global estimates for the water footprint of food, and an average shower length of 7 minutes with an inefficient shower head that uses 12 litres/min.) Hoekstra, A. (2012). *The hidden water resource use behind meat and dairy.* [online], Water Footprint Network. Available at: waterfootprint.org/media/downloads/Hoekstra-2012-Water-Meat-Dairy.pdf [Accessed 19 Aug 2016].

35 Greenpeace, (2009). *Amazon cattle footprint, Mato Grosso: State of destruction.* [online], Available at: www.greenpeace.org/international/en/publications/reports/amazon-cattle-footprint-mato/ [Accessed 21 Aug 2016].

36 Seeker, (2010). *Oceans' fish could disappear by 2050.* [online] Available at: www.seeker.com/oceans-fish-could-disappear-by-2050-1765058733.html#news.discovery.com [Accessed 20 Aug 2016].

37 Environmental Justice Foundation, (2003). *Squandering the Seas: How shrimp trawling is threatening ecological integrity and food security around the world.* London: Environmental Justice Foundation. Available at: ejfoundation.org/sites/default/files/public/squandering_the_seas.pdf [Accessed 20 Aug 2016].

38 CSIRO, (2005). *Balancing act: A triple bottom line analysis of the Australian economy. Volume 2.* [online] Available at: publications.csiro.au/rpr/download?pid=procite:ef189bac-499a-46db-be4d-b391a3cb05dc&dsid=DS2 [Accessed 20 Aug 2016].

39 World Health Organization, (2016). *Water-related diseases.* [online] Available at: www.who.int/water_sanitation_health/diseases/malnutrition/en/ [Accessed 20 Aug 2016].

40 Compassion in World Farming, (2004). *The global benefits of eating less meat.* [online] Available at: www.ciwf.org.uk/research/environment/the-global-benefits-of-eating-less-meat/ [Accessed 20 Aug 2016].

41 King, R. (2009). *4-a-week: Changing food consumption in the UK to benefit people and planet.* [online] Oxfam: Policy & Practice. Available at: policy-practice.oxfam.org.uk/publications/4-a-week-changing-food-consumption-in-the-uk-to-benefit-people-and-planet-114037 [Accessed 20 Aug 2016].

42 Vindas, M., Johansen, I., Folkedal, O., Höglund, E., Gorissen, M., Flik, G., Kristiansen, Ø. (2016). Brain serotonergic activation in growth-stunted farmed salmon: adaption versus pathology. [online] Available at: rsos.royalsocietypublishing.org/content/3/5/160030 [Accessed 4 Oct 2016]

43 Australian Bureau of Statistics, 2016, *Livestock Products, Australia*, cat. no. 7215.0. [online] Available at: www.abs.gov.au/AUSSTATS/abs@.nsf/mf/7215.0 [Accessed 4 Oct 2016] Also, IBISWorld, (2015). *Soaring seafood consumption fails to deliver significant growth for Australia's fishing and aquaculture industries.* [online] Available at: media.ibisworld.com.au/2015/12/15/soaring-seafood-consumption-fails-to-deliver-significant-growth-for-australias-fishing-and-aquaculture-industries/ [Accessed 4 Oct 2016]

44 Dietitians Association Australia, (2011). *A Guide to Vegan Eating.* [online] Available at: daa.asn.au/wp-content/uploads/2012/07/A-Guide-to-Vegan-Eating.pdf [Accessed 10 Nov 2016]. Also, American Dietetic Association, (2009). *Position of the American Dietetic Association: vegetarian diets.* [online] Volume 109 (7) 1266-82. Available at: www.ncbi.nlm.nih.gov/pubmed/19562864 [Accessed 10 Nov 2016].

45 National Health and Medical Research Council, (2013). *Eat for Health Australian Dietary Guidelines.* [online] Available at: www.eatforhealth.gov.au/sites/default/files/files/the_guidelines/n55a_australian_dietary_guidelines_summary_book.pdf [Accessed 10 Nov 2016].

46 Queensland Health Dietitian/Nutritionists, (2010). *Healthy eating for vegetarian pregnant & breastfeeding mothers.* [online] Available at: www.nevdgp.org.au/info/topics/maternity/antenatal_veget.pdf [Accessed 10 Nov 2016].

47 Leader, N., (2013). *Dietary Sources of Iron.* [online] Available at: www.seslhd.health.nsw.gov.au/rhw/Patient_Leaflets/Dietician/Pregnancy/Getting%20enough%20iron.pdf [Accessed 10 Nov 2016].

48 Dietitians Association Australia, (2011). *A Guide to Vegan Eating.* [online] Available at: daa.asn.au/wp-content/uploads/2012/07/A-Guide-to-Vegan-Eating.pdf [Accessed 10 Nov 2016].

49 ibid.

50 Queensland Health Dietitian/Nutritionists, (2010). *Healthy eating for vegetarian pregnant & breastfeeding mothers.* [online] Available at: www.nevdgp.org.au/info/topics/maternity/antenatal_veget.pdf [Accessed 10 Nov 2016].

51 Better Health Channel, (2012). *Vegetarian diets and children.* [online] Available at: www.betterhealth.vic.gov.au/health/healthyliving/vegetarian-diets-and-children [Accessed 10 Nov 2016].

52 Dietitians Association Australia, (2011). *A Guide to Vegan Eating.* [online] Available at: daa.asn.au/wp-content/uploads/2012/07/A-Guide-to-Vegan-Eating.pdf [Accessed 10 Nov 2016].

53 Greger (MD), M, (2016). *Calcium, Nutrition Facts* [online]. Available at: nutritionfacts.org/topics/calcium/ [Accessed 10 Nov 2016]

54 SELF Nutrition Data, n.d. *Molasses Nutrition Facts & Calories.* [online] Available at: nutritiondata.self.com/facts/sweets/5573/2 [Accessed 10 Nov 2016].

55 Greger (MD), M, (2014). *The Reason We Need More Antioxidants* [online]. Available at: nutritionfacts.org/2014/12/02/the-reason-we-need-more-antioxidants-and-why-were-not-getting-them/ [Accessed 10 Nov 2016]

Index

Our heartfelt thanks!

Every day we each have the power to have a positive impact with the food we choose to eat. So, we want to thank you for joining us on this journey to eat kindly, tread lightly and live well. One meal at a time you're making the world a better place.

We are so very grateful to everyone who contributed their recipes, talents, passion and support to make this cookbook possible. The world is more delightful and compassionate for having each of you in it.

We'd like to extend our heartfelt thanks to:

Our friends and family – for your love and support. With a special mention to those who contributed and tested recipes and those who assisted in many other important ways to this book: Tegan Steele, Joseph Bromley, Jenny Bromley, Rachel Armstrong, Shannon Driscoll, Sam Jankevics, Chris Bennett, Katie Walacavage, Fawn Porter, Raelene Govett, Phil Krzyska, Karen Bickley and Renee Wood.

Animals Australia's volunteers, donors and supporters – for sharing our vision of a kinder world and believing in us.

Our team – this book was a team effort and we're so grateful for your recipes, feedback, effort and enthusiasm. While many of our team contributed in many ways, a few people's remarkable contributions deserve a special mention. Isobel, your flare in the kitchen and passion for food took our recipes to the next level. Kat, your eye for the visual was invaluable. And Jodie, you were the glue that bound this book together.

The ABC Books team – for giving us the opportunity to share these recipes and tips. Especially, Jude McGee, for planting the seed for this cookbook and helping it to grow into what it is now; Barbara McClenahan, for your keen eye in editing and proofing; Katri Hilden, for help with the recipes; and the HarperCollins Design Studio, for bringing such a vibrant design to life.

Mercy For Animals and Physicians Committee for Responsible Medicine – for allowing us to adapt some of your resources.

Everyone who lent their talents to bring the photos in this book to life – Deborah Kaloper, Chris Middleton, Peta Grey, Hannah Kidd, Luke and Brooklyn from Brazen Models, Zoe and Barbara Payne, Victoria Martin and Hart&Co., and Carly at Establishment Studios.

Edgar's Mission Farm Sanctuary, Brightside Farm Sanctuary, Freedom Hill Sanctuary, Lefty's Place Sanctuary, Poplar Springs Animal Sanctuary – for allowing us to share the photos and stories of animals who are lucky enough to call your sanctuaries home. And to the photographers, Mark Peters, Tamara Kenneally and Kyle Behrand, for so beautifully capturing these animals and allowing us to use your photos. And also to Aussie Farms for allowing us to use your photos.

The talented and generous chefs whose recipes you can find in this book:

Bed & Broccoli – Nikki Medwell (bedandbroccoli.com.au)
hot for food (hotforfoodblog.com)
Melanie Baker, The Kind Cook (thekindcook.com)
Miriam Sorrell, author of Mouthwatering Vegan Recipes Book & Blog
    (mouthwateringvegan.com)
Rhea Parsons – The "V" Word (thevword.net)
Sam Turnbull (itdoesnttastelikechicken.com)
Suzy Spoon's Vegetarian Butcher (ssvb.com.au)
Tiahn Wright (tiahnwrite.com)
'What You Eat' Café (whatyoueat.com.au)

And finally, to Buddy, Nellie, Oscar, Nina, Tilly, Indie, Spice, Blue, Rusty, Mojo, Quincy, Bali and so many others. Your unconditional friendship and joy for life inspire us every day to make the world a better place for all living beings.

The ABC 'Wave' device is a trademark of the Australian Broadcasting Corporation and is used under licence by HarperCollins*Publishers* Australia.

First published in Australia in 2017
by HarperCollins*Publishers* Australia Pty Limited
ABN 36 009 913 517
harpercollins.com.au

HarperCollins*Publishers*
Level 13, 201 Elizabeth Street, Sydney, NSW 2000, Australia
Unit D1, 63 Apollo Drive, Rosedale, Auckland 0632, New Zealand
A 53, Sector 57, Noida, UP, India
1 London Bridge Street, London, SE1 9GF, United Kingdom
2 Bloor Street East, 20th floor, Toronto, Ontario M4W 1A8, Canada
195 Broadway, New York, NY 10007, USA

National Library of Australia Cataloguing-in-Publication entry:
    Title: Taste for life : eat kindly, tread lightly, live well /
    Animals Australia.
    ISBN: 9780733337895 (paperback)
    Notes: Includes index.
    Subjects: Plants, Edible.
    Vegetarian foods.
    Nutrition.
    Vegan cooking.
    Other Creators/Contributors:
    Animals Australia, author.
Dewey Number: 641.303

Cover and internal design: HarperCollins Design Studio
Cover images: Chris Middleton Photography
Food photography: Chris Middleton Photography
Styling: Deborah Kaloper
Internal picture credits: page 4 Mark Peters Photography, at Poplar Spring Animal Sanctuary. Republished under Creative Commons license. https://www.flickr.com/photos/markpetersphotography/15098939913/; 6–7 Chris Middleton Photography; 8 Yianni Aspradakis; 9 iStock; 11 Chris Middleton Photography; 14 iStock; 15 iStock; 17 iStock (top), Thinkstock (bottom); 19 iStock; 20 iStock; 21 Thinkstock; 22 Tamara Kenneally Photography (left), Aussie Farms (inset); 23 Freedom Hill Farm Sanctuary (top), Tamara Kenneally Photography (bottom); 24 Edgar's Mission Farm Sanctuary (top), Aussie Farms (top inset), Edgar's Mission Farm Sanctuary (bottom), Animals Australia (bottom inset); 25 David Fleetham/naturepl.com (top), Thinkstock (bottom); 28 Edgar's Mission Farm Sanctuary; 30 iStock; 31 Chris Bennett; 32 iStock; 33 iStock (top and bottom), Thinkstock (centre); 34 Chris Middleton Photography; 36 Shutterstock; 37 Shutterstock (top, centre below, bottom), iStock (centre above); 40 Edgar's Mission Farm Sanctuary; 42–49 Chris Middleton Photography; 52 Shutterstock (top left and right, bottom left), Thinkstock (bottom right), iStock (top left), Shutterstock (top right, bottom left and right); 54–56 iStock and Shutterstock; 59 iStock; 61 Shutterstock; 62 Shutterstock; 63 Thinkstock and iStock.

Printed and bound in China by RR Donnelley
Printed on 100% recycled paper